Modern Bride®

Just Married

Also available from Wiley's *Modern Bride*® Library:

Modern Bride® Wedding Celebrations
The Complete Wedding Planner for Today's Bride
by Cele Goldsmith Lalli and Stephanie H. Dahl

Modern Bride® Guide to Etiquette
Answers to the Questions Today's Couples Really Ask
by Cele Goldsmith Lalli

Modern Bride®
Just Married

Everything you need to know
to plan your new life together

STEPHANIE H. DAHL

John Wiley & Sons, Inc.
New York • Chichester • Brisbane • Toronto • Singapore

Library of Congress Cataloging-in-Publication Data:

Dahl, Stephanie H.
    Modern bride just married: everything you need to know to plan your new
    life together/Stephanie H. Dahl.
        p.   cm.
    Includes bibliographical references and index.
    ISBN 0–471–59669–8 (paper)
    1. Marriage—United States. 2. Man-woman relationships—United States.
    3. Intimacy (Psychology) I. Modern bride. II. Title.
    HQ734 IN PROCESS
    646.7'8--dc20   93-48959

To my husband, Clifford,
who has helped me learn how to live, and grow, in love.
Happy Anniversary!

PREFACE

For all that can be said about marriage, only one thing is certain: if a couple can't change and grow together, they will certainly change and grow apart. Love relationships are never static. Either they move forward, generating continuous self-discovery and mutual satisfaction, or they stall, stagnate, and wither away. People committed to long-term relationships expect some sidestepping and backsliding here and there, but they never lose sight of the forward momentum they must maintain, and they never take for granted the privilege, and the power, the gift of love bestows.

This learning and loving and changing and growing make marriage a dynamic, dramatic process, one that begins to unfold the very first day of your new life together as husband and wife, and one that continues each and every day of your life thereafter. It takes skill to manage living intimately in process. The attitudes and behaviors necessary to sustain a lifelong commitment can be developed, but they don't always come easily, or naturally. We are, after all, only human. I sincerely believe, however, that if more people worked at their marriages, then more marriages would work, and work well.

What I'm talking about is not just a lasting marriage, but a good one, a fulfilling one, a joyful one. That kind of marriage has always been the ideal, and maybe it was always hard to achieve, but it's probably harder than ever now. For one thing, there are fewer and fewer intact families, and thus fewer and fewer good marriage models for newlyweds to emulate. For another, the character traits promoted and encouraged as everyday "survival skills" in an aggressive, competitive society are decidedly at odds with such attributes as patience, trust, and self-sacrifice, the qualities that are needed to establish and maintain a loving partnership at home.

Frankly, it's time for a change, in marriage, in the family, and in society, and today's just-married couples are the ones who can make it. You are not naive. You are older and wiser, and maybe a bit relationship-weary yourselves, so you know what's at stake and how much you have to gain by making this one work. You've entered the contract freely, out of choice, and out of love. Now you have to make the romance real by working on the friendship.

I've done a lot of things in my life that I'm proud of, but what I've done best, and what's brought out the best in me, is my marriage. And this from a person who never intended to marry in the first place, much less spend her professional life writing about it! Like many of you, I imagine, I was raised by a single parent (my husband was too), so I didn't grow up with a marriage model. Once married, I moved clear across the country, from Texas to New York, to begin a new life, so I never had the abiding support of old friends and family members to help me adjust. And, like so many of today's couples, my husband Clifford and I had mostly our differences in common, differences in religion, politics, age, and regional/cultural backgrounds. Yet, we made our marriage work by learning to rely on each other first and foremost, and by bringing some common sense to the commitment we had made.

This year, we happily and gratefully celebrate our 25th wedding anniversary. Much of what we've learned about marriage has been self-taught, as we met each new challenge. It's an ongoing process of learning and adapting. I don't have a magic formula for "happily ever after." Nobody does. But I do believe in marriage as a workable, rewarding, redeeming way of life, and I believe that lasting love and happiness are more than just matters of luck.

Modern Bride® *Just Married* is based on those beliefs. The book begins when the real work of marriage begins—right after the return from the honeymoon. The predictable areas of adjustment in married life, in-laws or sex or money, are arranged roughly in the order in which you're likely to encounter them, but the book doesn't have to be read in sequence. Rather, the chapters are divided, and indexed, so that you can refer to them again and again, just as you would consult a trusted friend, whenever the need arises.

In writing this book, I've not only drawn on my own marital experience to guide you through any difficulties, but I've also listened to the lessons of other couples, and consulted experts for help with professional matters. This is a book that invites communication and cooperation, and I hope the two of you will use it that way. I also hope you'll take advantage of the many resources offered in the Appendix for further information on various topics.

Now that you are committed to a mutually responsible, lifetime partnership, you have to learn how to make good on that commitment. You can do that by being kind to each other, by listening to your head *and* your heart, and by renewing your promise to each other over and over again, every day if necessary.

Marriage makes magic in your soul. Believe it. Work for it. And, be assured that it's worth all the effort.

Stephanie H. Dahl

ACKNOWLEDGMENTS

For their time in interviews and their help in gathering information, sincere appreciation goes to the following: Don Badders; Terry Barnett, Esq.; Laurie Bergman; Phyllis Bernstein; Dawn and Gary Bivona; Elizabeth Erwin Blackman, Ph.D.; Jonathan Brenner; Nancy Brett; Bonnie and Michael Brodowski; Claire and Charlie Casey; Stephanie and Victor Cassone; Clare Castaldo; Charles Cole, Ph.D.; Rev. Mark Connolly; Paul Dasher, Ph.D.; Jodie Davis; Susan Deguzman; Steve Dixon; Maria Ecks-Chamberlain; Rabbi Charles Familant; Florence Foelak; Dena and Billy Gambino; Jane W. Glander, Esq.; John Gottman, Ph.D.; Clara Grandy; Steve Greene; Christine Grillo; Rosa Lee Harker; Joan C. Hawxhurst; Colleen and Phil Hayes; Susan Hefner; Harville Hendrix, Ph.D.; Leland J. Hoch; Katherine Hoffman; Molly Holmes; Tim Hozen; Joanne Johnson; Phil Kibak; Claudia and Roy Loomis; Chris Martin; Jennifer and Angus McCullock; Stella McGuire; Ray McNally; Diahann and Jay Menachem; John Money, M.D.; Adam Morgan, Esq.; Robert W. Nightengale, Jr.; Alisa Parcells; Jim Prucha; Joy Purcell; Cathleen and Kevin Rahimzadeh; Helen and Richard Rauch; Thomas W. Roberts, Ph.D.; Kari Rustici; Justin O. Schechter, M.D.; Ed Schilling, III; Ken Scott; Gale A. Sloan, R.N.; Karen W. Spero; Gary Stanek; Karen and Jeff Stelmach; Deborah Vinnick Tesler, M.D. and Peter Tesler, M.D.; Susan Tew; Annie Thurow; Anne Tobin-Ashe, Ph.D.; Marv Tuttle; Charles White; Alexandra White-Ritchie; Emily and Scott Whitman; Amy Winkelman, Esq.; Stephanie and Chris Winter; and Patricia Magloire Wolfe.

For their help as expert consultants on specialized chapters, I am extremely grateful to: Lloyd Benson, CPA, PFS, CFP; Sarah Eldrich, Esq.; Agnes A. Roach, CFP; Judy Seifer, Ph.D.; and Leonard Vinnick, M.D.

For helping me make this the best book it could be, I am especially indebted to Cele Goldsmith Lalli, my mentor, my friend, and my editor at *Modern Bride;* to Judith N. McCarthy, herself a newlywed and my editor at John Wiley & Sons; and to my son, Aaron H. Dahl, my resident artist and assistant.

CONTENTS

Foreword by Cele Lalli *xiii*

FOREWORD

I travel a lot talking with engaged women, particularly at the *Modern Bride* store shows held in the gift registry at department and specialty stores throughout the country. Often these women are accompanied by recently married friends. These newlyweds tell me that after the excitement of organizing their wedding, when the magazine and the wedding planning books were like personal advisors consulted daily, there is then a void. Just when they need to be buoyed up in what is for many newlyweds a postwedding blues period, they have nowhere to turn to help them deal with the reality of life after the honeymoon. That void is now filled with the book in your hand.

Just Married is an essential reference and resource for adapting to marriage. It will help you handle every aspect of your personal partnership as well as family, business, and social interaction. Because regardless of how close you've been throughout your dating and engagement, life *does* change after the wedding.

Through focus groups with recently married couples, we know what questions, conflicts, and adjustments are uppermost in your minds. With rare exceptions, you will be facing difficult challenges inherent in living together as a married couple. You will be grateful to know that you are not alone. This book enables you to identify and define these challenges as they affect your relationship and to learn from the experiences of others how to cope constructively. It is your guide to successful living and loving in the first few years of marriage. With a firm foundation, the rest of your lives should be a piece of wedding cake.

Cele G. Lalli
Editor-in-Chief
Modern Bride

CHAPTER 1

Crossing the Threshold

*I*t's Monday morning after the honeymoon. You lie there listening to the in-cessant buzz of the alarm, wondering how long your husband, your *new* hus-band, will let it blare before he shuts it off. This is it, you realize: the first regu-lar day of the rest of your life as a married couple.

After all the planning, all the excitement, and all the fanfare, this day brings with it a new anticipation. Are you any different now than you were a couple of weeks ago? Have changes taken place between the two of you already? What's next? You wonder.

You go to work, and everyone asks you about the honeymoon. "Where did you stay? Was it romantic? When did you get back?" they want to know. Those who were at the wedding tell you what a wonderful time they had, how radi-ant you looked, and how beautifully everything was done. Someone even tells you how fabulous you look now, thus concluding that marriage evidently agrees with you. "Thank you," you answer. "Yes, I think it does."

But then, before you know it, this very new newlywed phase is over, too. The congratulatory comments from friends and colleagues cease, you two stop talking so much about the wedding and the honeymoon, and the patterns and pressures of daily living slowly, but surely, start to assert themselves. Reality sets in.

This recognition comes in different ways at different times for different rea-sons, but it always comes. For some, it arrives gradually as everyday routines dis-place romantic serendipity; for others, reality hits in a flash, prompted by a heap of wet towels on the floor or an intrusive telephone call from an interfering in-law. Regardless of when or how it happens, though, there is always a tinge of sadness, not because the reality is so bad, but because those totally unrealistic notions about the perfect partner and the perfect married life, maybe even the perfect self, have to be abandoned.

Waking up to those realities requires a process of adjusting attitudes and be-haviors, and that's exactly what the newlywed stage provides—a period of ad-justment. During the first three years or so of marriage, the two of you will con-tinue to discover wondrous new things about each other, while also working to redefine yourselves in light of this new arrangement. You will laugh and cry and fight and make up and be sure and uncertain at the same time, all in an attempt to strike the magic balance between romance and reality.

For some of you, the ones with the truest love and the deepest determina-tion, the scales will always tip, be it ever so slightly, in favor of your hearts, so

---

꧁ DO YOU SEE YOURSELF HERE? ꧂

- Do you feel neglected, and wonder why your spouse isn't as attentive as he or she was on the honeymoon?
- Do you have moments of loneliness, even when your spouse is around?
- Do you feel as though, now that all the excitement is over, you have nothing much to look forward to?
- Do you occasionally feel "homesick" for your parents, your old friends, your old way of life?
- Do you feel overwhelmed, and disillusioned, by how much work it is to meet the multiple demands of home, family, friends, job, etc.?
- Have you made some unpleasant discoveries about your spouse?
- Are you surprised by the amount of bickering and nitpicking you've fallen into?
- Do memories of your honeymoon, good or bad, haunt the present in an unproductive way?
- Do you feel down sometimes, for reasons you can't quite identify?

The more "yes" answers you have, the more you need to read on.

---

that the weight of even the harshest realities will seem somehow easier to bear. And you will become the lucky ones, the ones for whom the honeymoon goes on forever.

The Honeymoon Hangover

"Our honeymoon was so perfect," Janice says. "We went to Bermuda and it rained for nine out of ten days. Now that may sound crazy, but to me, it was perfect. We didn't feel we had to go anywhere or do anything; we were just alone, together, 100 percent of the time, day and night. It was so romantic."

It's a Sunday afternoon about seven months after the wedding. Janice is eager to talk because she's home alone, as she is every Sunday afternoon because her husband works weekends.

"I'll tell you, though," she continues, "it doesn't take long to know the honeymoon's over." She shakes her head and sighs. "This business of me working Monday through Friday and Jerry working Wednesday through Sunday has put a real strain on our marriage already."

Janice confesses that she was unreasonable about how much togetherness she expected at first. "I'd wait for him to get home to do even the simplest things, like running down to the grocery or going to get gas," she says, "and I'd get upset if he went anywhere or did anything at all without me. I thought marriage was about being together *all* the time, like our honeymoon was, and since our work schedules limited our time together, I became overly jealous and possessive of whatever free time we did have."

Soon, Jerry began to feel suffocated as Janice felt more neglected. Arguments erupted before a discussion ensued. Now, the two are trying to deal with the routine, and the restrictions, of their daily schedules. But it still isn't always easy. Janice admits to feeling lonely sometimes, particularly on the weekends, and Jerry feels guilty just going out for a beer with friends after work. "But I was making us both crazy, so I knew I had to get over the togetherness thing. I mean, this is real life, and life isn't one big romance novel. We do have to work for a living." Janice pauses, then adds, "I guess I just hate to admit that the honeymoon is over."

Sometimes the honeymoon can be too perfect, thereby setting up unreasonable expectations for life after the couple gets home. Whether it's dancing till dawn, nonstop lovemaking, or indulgence in luxury, the conditions and behaviors of this one special trip are not likely to continue forever. The honeymoon is not really the beginning of the marriage; rather, it is a transition period between the ritual of the wedding and the reality of life to come.

Honeymoon Regrets

Couples have to forgive themselves for being only human on their honeymoons, especially if something happens to mar the anticipated perfection they'd always dreamed of.

Such was the case for Cheryl and Paul. The two were tired. They had a huge wedding, then made a long flight to reach their honeymoon destination. When they finally arrived and were shown to what they had thought would be a luxury suite, at least by the reputation of the hotel and the price they were paying, Cheryl couldn't contain herself. "This place is the pits," she pronounced. "I refuse to spend my honeymoon in such a room!"

It was the couple's first fight, ever. "Paul had made all the arrangements," she explains, "and so he took what I said as a personal affront. The more he accused me of overreacting, the more determined I became to change rooms. He wouldn't see to it, so I did. Then it boiled down to which was more important, our being together or my having luxury accommodations?"

Paul and Cheryl have been married six months now, but they still talk about that awful argument and feel regret that it haunts the memory of what should have been an idyllic week together. "It's interesting, though," Cheryl admits. "The arguments we've had since stem from the same problem: Paul says I overreact, and I say he reads too much into what comes out of my mouth. Maybe we'll come to understand each other better so we can have a perfect second honeymoon."

The honeymoon is a time for a couple to revel in each other without the demands and distractions of daily life, and that is supposed to be a delightful, if somewhat unreal, experience. But regardless of whether your honeymoon met your expectations, exceeded them, or fell short, the memory of it all has to be put in perspective. You can help each other do that by talking about what went right, and wrong, with your trip, by keeping some of the honeymoon lessons in mind when planning future vacations, and by sharing honeymoon stories, especially the funny ones, with other newlywed couples. (No doubt you'll be surprised by the similarities of your experiences.)

Years from now, you'll laugh when you recall the nervousness and the blunders, even the silly misunderstandings. And, when the going gets tough, you'll also recall the passion and the promise you felt in those just-married days. And you'll rely on loving honeymoon memories to sustain you through the romantic history the two of you share.

Postwedding Blues

For months, probably a year or more, you and your fiancé were extremely busy and very excited. There was so much going on: planning the wedding, managing myriad details, communicating with family and friends, attending parties, writing notes and making phone calls, deciding on a honeymoon destination, finding a place to live, choosing home furnishings—what a whirlwind! The list of things to do went on and on.

And then the wedding day arrived and you were at the apex of attention, the ones on whom all eyes rested and to whom all efforts were devoted. It was thrilling, it was heady, it was a dream come true.

Suddenly, it was over. You were whisked away on a honeymoon that was restful, romantic, and fun, but even then the reality of life after the wedding began to creep into your consciousness. Once back home, it really was all over. The moments for which you had worked, planned, and dreamed had come and gone.

Psychologists tell us that a letdown in mood, even some temporary depression, is perfectly normal after periods of hyperactivity and events colored by high anticipation. A well-documented example of this is the postpartum depression routinely experienced by new mothers after the birth of their babies, but amazingly similar downswings in emotion are also reported by athletes after championship games are played, artists after major works are completed, and even business executives after performance goals are reached. It is as though the human spirit temporarily deflates once all that focused energy is spent, and a period of quiet contemplation, sometimes perceived as sadness, is needed for rejuvenation and renewal before an overall sense of well-being can return.

Periods of postwedding blues can also be triggered by very real circumstances that might leave one feeling vulnerable. Homesickness for family and friends, job changes or an inability to find work in a new locale, worries about money or health, or plain physical exhaustion—any one of these might be the culprit.

Don't let the postwedding blues get you down for long. To hasten the return of your usual, good-natured self, try these common antidotes for depression:

•   Embark upon a new project, like decorating a room or refinishing furniture, or resurrect an old hobby, like painting or needlework.

- Make a point to get out more socially and to spend more time with happy friends you enjoy.
- Plan a special weekend getaway with your spouse.
- Read uplifting books and see light movies.
- Do something that will make you feel good about yourself: perform some charitable work, get a new hairdo, complete a chore you've been putting off.
- Get enough rest.
- Exercise regularly to release those endorphins!

If down moods persist and deepen into what you consider a real depression, or if you've become unusually irritable or argumentative, see your doctor. There could be physiological reasons for the way you're feeling, including hormonal changes caused by the use of oral contraceptives. (See Chapters 5 and 11 for more information.)

The Weird Period

"I'm just back from the honeymoon and people are saying to me, 'So, how's married life?' How am I supposed to know? I'm married a week and the whole time maids have been cooking and cleaning for me while I'm living it up in luxury. Nobody knows anything at that stage."

Stacy, 26, married Jonathan, 32, after a traditional, two-year courtship that did not include cohabitation. Both share almost identical family backgrounds; both are of the same religious faith; and both come from within blocks of each other in Queens, New York. They are best friends, and they never had a major disagreement before the wedding. But then they got married.

"It was like from the moment the honeymoon was over, the honeymoon was over," Stacy says. "It was the weirdest thing. In fact, we call it our 'weird period,' that first six months of our marriage when we almost broke up. It was awful. We fought about every little thing, stupid things, like buying new throw pillows or using each other's towels or talking on the telephone. I couldn't believe it, even though I did it. The bickering and fighting got so bad that, by four months, I really didn't think we were going to make it. That's when we got the names of some counselors."

With the help of supportive families and a dedicated effort at building listening and communication skills, Stacy and Jonathan managed to list five issues that consistently generated problems between them:

1. Although they had spent an enormous amount of time together during the courtship, the couple had not really discussed the day-to-day realities of their new life together after the marriage.
2. Their parents, mainly her family, had given them a large, traditional wedding, and had made most of the arrangements. Stacy and Jonathan hadn't been terribly involved, although they had had a few spats over minor wedding-related details, which both attributed to prewedding jitters.

3. After the marriage, Stacy moved out of her father's large house and into her husband's small apartment, where he had been living as a bachelor for several years. There was no room for her stuff, and her attempts to rearrange things and to make a home were seen as intrusive.
4. Jonathan has many hobbies and interests, some of which, like tennis or basketball, he routinely enjoys with friends. Stacy had no outside interests to occupy her own time.
5. Jonathan started a new business right after they got married. Stacy had never worried about money before, so the financial uncertainty and strict budgeting made her uncomfortable.

After making the preliminary list, Stacy and Jonathan then looked beneath the surface issues to the real source of conflict. The list started to look like this:

1. No substantive discussions before the marriage = idealized notions of what married life would be like.
2. Wedding-related spats = the beginning of what Jonathan perceived as a loyalty issue over Stacy's alliance with her parents.
3. Moving to Jonathan's apartment = a very real space problem and no sense of a shared home.
4. Outside interests = a feeling of loneliness and abandonment, even jealousy of Jonathan's friends on Stacy's part.
5. New business = a stressor at any time, but especially so at this stage, because Stacy obviously expected her husband to provide the same financial security that her father had.

This look at their adjustment list is instructive because problems like these are extremely common during the first few months of marriage. It is a stressful period because the basic issues between you—marital roles, expectations, money, sex, in-laws—all begin to surface, but you don't yet have the strategies in place to deal with them. Sometimes, as with Stacy and Jonathan, it takes a while even to recognize what the issues really are.

Hence, a "weird period" ensues in which neither partner really acts like his or her old self, and during which both probably question the future stability of the marriage, even if they don't express it. In any event, both definitely feel that the honeymoon is, indeed, over.

A little over a year later, Stacy announces that "things are wonderful." The couple has moved into a bigger apartment; Stacy is taking sewing lessons; Jonathan's business is going well; the couple has set some short-term goals for the future; and they have learned to talk about, rather than shout about, topics that concern them. Best of all, calm and confidence have returned to their relationship. "The honeymoon may be over," Stacy says, smiling, "but the romance isn't."

It doesn't have to be for you either. If you find yourself in a "weird period" of your own, see if you can generate a list of the biggest problems between you. If you can't do it yourselves, get a neutral friend or relative, or a counseling professional, to help you. Then, examine the list, talk about what's really at issue, and look for possible solutions together. (See more about conflict and communication in the next chapter.)

Stacy and Jonathan took a day off from work to stay home and talk through their list. They began with breakfast in bed and allowed no interruptions from the telephone or the doorbell. They laughed and cried, and talked, all day long. Most of all, they reaffirmed their love and commitment to each other.

So, the message is this: Don't panic! Lots of couples go through rocky periods of initial adjustment, but then go on to enjoy loving, lasting marriages. You can too.

Small Adjustments

Modern Bride's ongoing Consumer Council studies reveal that the average age of a couple at first marriage is currently 26.1 years for the bride and 28.6 years for the groom. What does that mean for the marriage?

On the plus side, it means that today's couples are more mature personally, more established in the workplace, and probably more experienced in interpersonal relationships than they used to be. They are also likely to have been living on their own for a while before they got married. That could be a negative, at least in terms of the small personal adjustments they will have to make. Old habits die hard, and the more firmly entrenched they are, the more difficult they are to change.

No matter how well you think you know someone, the small revelations of actually living together always come as a surprise. Luckily, the "honeymoon spirit" that reigns over the first few months can help ease the shock, sometimes. When that fails, maybe you can rely on good old common sense.

"I'm a morning person and Sally is a night person," says Joseph, now married five months. "It never occurred to me that that would translate into my reading the newspaper with my coffee in the kitchen every morning, and her reading it in bed every night. Did you ever try to get to sleep while someone next to you is crinkling and crumpling a newspaper? Let me tell you, it isn't easy."

Sally and Joseph dated for five years before their marriage and so they thought they knew each other pretty well, even though they did not cohabit before the wedding. "We agree on all the big things, our values and beliefs," he says, "so I simply saw our personal habits as complementary: she's a little disorganized, I'm neat; she likes to take her time, I like to get things done right away; she loves pets in the house, I like pet rocks. You know, the usual opposite attraction kind of thing. . . ."

Opposites may attract, but they don't necessarily complement. The different talents and skills each partner brings to a relationship provide a complementary balance only when they are perceived as adding to the overall strength of the relationship. For example, one partner loves working outdoors while the other prefers inside chores, or one partner is adept at entertaining while the other is a bit reticent or shy. When different skills and habits are not seen as assets to the partnership, however, they can easily become sources of conflict.

Sally and Joseph value each other's different strengths and have a sense of humor about their different weaknesses. Because they know each other so well, they have been able to talk about their personal habits and routines and to make some compromises out of consideration for each other. "After all, it's usually not a matter of right or wrong, good or bad," says Joseph. "It's simply that two people are different and they do things in different ways."

During their courtship, including periods of cohabitation before the wedding, couples tend to idealize each other as the beloved and to willingly overlook minor faults and quirks. They also try to remain on their own best courtship behaviors. The old joke that ends with the punch line, "Why get married and ruin the relationship?" alludes to a common experience: once the thrill of the chase is over and the lifelong commitment is made, spouses become themselves, which means they are less mindful of their own behavior and more critical of each other's.

Awareness of self and consideration for the other are vital to making small personal adjustments to your spouse; they may be integral to larger adjustments as well. Marriage and family specialists consistently point to the couple's "adaptability factor" as a key ingredient for marital stability and success. After all, the reasoning goes, if two people aren't versatile enough to adapt to each other's small idiosyncrasies, how will they ever be able to negotiate the bigger differences that may arise between them?

Socks on the floor, clutter on the counter, hair in the sink, potato chips in bed—pick your pet peeve, but don't pick on everything. People do not change behaviors because of nagging and criticism; they change because they are motivated to do so out of consideration for the other, and because that other has the ability to express a need for change in a kind, constructive way. When you can accept your spouse as the person he or she really is, along with all the weaknesses and foibles of being human, then you know you're on your way to a mature and lasting love.

Defining Expectations

Why did the two of you get married? What benefits do you expect from married life? What kind of spouse did you think your mate would be? What kind of spouse are you? What kind of couple?

You will ask yourself questions like these more than once in the first months of marriage, maybe even more than once a day when things are really going badly and you're really doubting yourself. But take heart: all couples go through this sort of questioning and second-guessing because all couples come to marriage with certain expectations of how it will be. The newlywed period could be called an ongoing reality check.

Disparities between expectations before the marriage and realities after the fact become apparent pretty fast, and although they may not all be major surprises, even little picky things can take some getting used to. Obviously, the greater and more serious the expectations gap, the greater the number of adjustments that will have to be made, probably on both sides.

What Other Couples Say . . .

Ironically, couples who expect to face major adjustments, and who talk about and plan for them beforehand, often report that the early months of marital adjustment turn out to be easier than they had anticipated. Conversely, couples who thought marriage would relieve some of the stresses between them and make life simpler often discover that the day-to-day adjustments present more of a challenge than they had expected.

And then there are those pleasant surprises, which may necessitate an adjustment of a different kind. "The nicest thing about marriage is that it's so . . . well . . . nice!" remarks Sara, now married two years. "I mean, our relationship is so warm and comforting, and I'm just amazed at how happy I am. I didn't grow up around any good marriages, so to me, this is just almost too good to be true. I've had to learn to trust happiness, to decide that I deserve it."

Sara's comments indicate some fundamental truths about marital expectations:

1. Our earliest image of what marriage is supposed to be like comes from the models we experience through our own parents and families.
2. Everyone has to take responsibility for his or her own happiness.
3. One has to believe that he or she is worthy of being happy and being loved.

Depending on the models we've had and our own self-esteem, we will create marital expectations that are unrealistically high or low, which will then cause a more difficult period of adjustment, or we will arrive at expectations that are reasonably realistic. Even when realistic, however, it is unlikely that both partners will have an identical set of marital images.

So, some fine-tuning and minor adjustments are to be expected in the early stages of your new partnership. Rare is the couple who is so perfectly "in synch" that virtually no marital adjustments are needed. Even newlyweds who have lived together previously can't assume that their minor marital adjustments are over. "We lived together for three years before the wedding," says one newlywed, "but we didn't share our bank accounts until after we were legally married. Wow. What revelations that prompted, for both of us!"

This is marriage, and funny things happen to a couple after they've said "I do."

Redefining Yourselves

Some argue that any expectation of marriage based on the past is bound to be unrealistic and inappropriate because family life has changed so rapidly with each generation that today's couples simply have no relevant models to follow.

They point to the high divorce rates, blended and stepfamilies, and single-parent homes of the previous generation and make dire predictions about today's newlyweds and the future of the American family.

Not necessarily. Don't let doomsday theorists create a self-fulfilling prophecy for you! If you or your spouse is the child of divorce, or the product of an unhappy or abusive home, don't automatically assume that your own marriage is doomed when you have your first spat or face your first difficult adjustment. A lot of couples interviewed for this book expressed concern about their own less-than-ideal family backgrounds, not realizing that an awareness of the mistakes of one's parents is the first step toward creating more positive patterns for one's self.

Certainly, if either of you has serious scars from your childhood or some as yet unresolved issues between you and your parents, you might consider getting professional help to put the hurt to rest so you can get on with the rest of your life. You don't want others' mistakes to blight your own potential for personal happiness.

Dr. Anne Tobin-Ashe, a well-known family therapist and clinical staff member at the Georgetown (University) Family Center, emphasizes that each generation of couples has its work cut out for it. The World War II generation struggled toward economic security, while their children, the Baby Boomers, raised consciousness and asserted individuality. "The work of today's generation of newlyweds is to achieve an emotional stability in the home," she says. "I'm optimistic, because I see it happening already. As women have taken on more roles for themselves, men have begun to realize that they, too, are multidimensional."

Multiple roles mean more equity between the partners and a fuller participation in the marriage for both the man and the woman. "The best way to realize your expectations of marriage is by reducing the expectations of your partner and increasing the expectations of yourself," Dr. Ashe advises. That way, marriage becomes less of a 50/50 equation and more of a 100 percent proposi-

---

Affirming Each Other

Some couples have difficulty completing these statements. Why don't you give it a try, then use them again and again as a way of reaffirming and rearticulating your commitment to each other.

1.   The reason we got married was . . .
2.   The reason we'll stay married is . . .
3.   Three to five years from now, we expect to be . . .
4.   Our most immediate goal is to . . .
5.   The greatest strength we have as a couple is our . . .
6.   The thing I love most about my spouse is his or her . . .
7.   One couple whose marriage we both admire is . . .

tion in which both partners give their all to accept and adapt to each other, to identify and build on their combined strengths, and to work together to achieve mutual goals that include a lasting, loving marriage.

Setting Precedents

While working to modify and adjust the initial expectations each of you has brought to the marriage, you'll also have to be careful not to replace them with new ones that are equally unrealistic or difficult to sustain. Take the new wife who is so anxious to ingratiate herself with her mother-in-law that she agrees, Sunday after Sunday at first, to go to her in-laws' house for dinner. Pretty soon, a pattern is established and an expectation is set.

Eventually, though, the Sunday comes when the now not-so-new wife wants to go somewhere else for dinner, or to just stay at home. She demands to know why she and her husband have to go to her mother-in-law's every week, and she hears, "Because we always do and we always have."

It doesn't take long for "always" to become forever. Whether you're talking about where you spend major holidays or who picks up dirty socks, expectations born out of regular routines are all too easy to establish, and oh so difficult to undo. So here's a simple rule that can make a lifetime of difference in your marriage: *Don't set any precedents you don't intend to keep.*

That rule has to be applied to each other as well as to family members. It is perhaps a little easier to be vigilant and to say "no" to others, relatives or friends, because you don't live with them and they're not the primary objects of your affection. But consciously setting limits or saying "no" to your spouse can be a real challenge, especially in the newlywed period when you are naturally inclined to do every little thing you can to please and delight your beloved.

It may sound cold and unromantic to talk about the bargains that are struck between two people in marriage, but that's exactly what takes place because that's what marriage is: a partnership of give and take. Some agreements will be even trade-offs of the "I'll do this if you'll do that" variety; others will be special favors, a "just this once" kind of offer. Even or lopsided, large or small, the point is not about keeping score, but about each partner feeling satisfied overall, and neither one growing resentful of any agreements, tacit or expressed, they have made.

On a larger scale, what we're really talking about are two fundamentally different approaches to building a lifetime relationship. The choice is yours: you can either (a) start working on your marriage right away by making conscious choices and discussing any differences between you, thereby minimizing the potential for future problems; or, (b) make light of your differences, let things slide, and try to postpone dealing with issues until there is a major problem. Frankly, if you've chosen b, you're asking for trouble.

It may not be easy to say, "Honey, I love you, but I'm not ironing all those cotton shirts," but you have to make yourself say it if you don't want to iron those shirts for the rest of your life. And ironing shirts really isn't a *big* thing. You can probably put off confrontations about laundry for quite a while, and then just blithely announce one day that, from here on out, all cotton shirts are going to the cleaner's.

But what about the bigger issues? What about the man who can't deal with his own mother or family, and so constantly tries to foist the emotional burden of all of them onto you? However difficult it might have been to say that you were through ironing shirts, it will be ten times harder to say, "Honey, I love you, but you're going to have to deal with your mother yourself."

We all have limits to what we're willing to accept for a lifetime. From household chores to family relationships to marital roles, the more honest you are about yours, and the sooner, the better off you both will be.

The Domestic Scene

Most likely the inventory on the next page will show some discrepancies, and the list of chores for the woman will be longer than for the man. Don't worry; you're perfectly normal—unfortunately. Check out this statistic from the *Journal of Marriage and the Family*:

> Virtually every study [done in the last 10 years] investigating the division of household labor has come to two basic conclusions: women perform approximately twice as much labor as men; and women perform *qualitatively* different types of chores than men (Blair & Johnson, 570).

Or, to put it another way that might have more immediate meaning: Who makes your bed in the morning?

We all know about women's work and men's work and all the drudgery in between, but the truly amazing thing is how firmly entrenched these stereotypes are and how they reassert themselves into the lives of even the most enlightened couples. The division of household labor along gender lines might have been reasonable before women went out to work in such massive numbers. These days, though, when 72 percent of all married women between the ages of 25 and 44 work to help bring home the bacon, it's only fair that their husbands be expected to help cook it and serve it up!

"Tony is pretty good about helping out around the house," Diane says. "I mean, he takes care of all the yardwork and stuff, but he'll even run the vacuum or throw in a load of laundry when I ask him to, and we do the grocery shopping and other errands together on Saturday mornings."

Tony and Diane have been married two years and both work full-time. Thus, the laundry, cleaning, bill paying, and other indoor chores get done on weeknights after dinner, which Diane usually cooks and Tony usually cleans up, and the shopping, yardwork, and other outdoor chores and special projects are left for the weekends. The division of labor in the couple's home is generally allocated along traditional gender lines, not so much because they believe in rigid sexual stereotypes, but because "it just works out that way." At least there is a division of labor, and Tony and Diane seem reasonably happy with their arrangement.

Domestic Bliss

Here's a fun exercise. Go down this list together and check the column you agree on.

Who "Should" ...	Man	Woman	Either
wash cars			
wash dishes			
cook meals			
barbecue outside			
vacuum floors			
shampoo carpets			
get car serviced			
pump gas			
drive (when both are in car)			
weed flower beds			
mow lawn			
mop floors			
clean toilets			
water plants			
clip shrubbery			
feed pets			
repair a faucet			
pay the bills			
do the taxes			
make dinner reservations			
go grocery shopping			
invite guests over			
plan menus			
set the dinner table			
buy holiday gifts			
write thank-you notes			
send greeting cards			
do laundry			
drop off cleaning			
buy wines and liquors			
iron			
make the bed			
wash windows			
paint a room			
clean out the garage			
make more money			
change diapers			
call babysitters			

Now go back through the list using a different color pen and mark each chore not by who "should" do it, but by who does do it in your home. Any discrepancies between what you do and what you believe? Is the list lopsided? What do you think that means? Read on.

"My father never did a thing around the house, not a blessed thing," Diane says. "Sure, he put in long hours at the plant, but my mother always had paid jobs, too, and still she did everything at home, plus raise us kids, and spoil Dad rotten. I swore I'd never live that way, so I guess I'm lucky to have found the guy I did."

Is This Domestic Bliss?

Tony and Diane are typical of so many couples in so many ways that her comments are worth reviewing for some of the troublesome facts, and fallacies, about domestic life. First of all, she says that Tony "helps out" around the house, implying that the house is her primary responsibility and that his contributions are strictly voluntary. Of course, he does do "yardwork and stuff," the man's work, which is more than her father did.

Diane's description of her father as someone who "never did a thing" and her mother as the one who did it all, and spoiled him on top of it, gets at a fundamental problem for today's couples: there aren't a lot of role models to follow regarding equitable divisions of labor in the home. Younger men aren't likely to have seen their fathers in very many domestic roles, but young women are likely to have grown up with some version of a supermom.

Finally, although Diane swore she'd "never live that way," her step forward doesn't seem to have been exactly a giant one. Behavior always lags behind ideology, and progress from one generation to the next, in anything, is slow and meager. Even so, maybe if Diane relied less on being "lucky" and more on expressing rightful expectations, Tony would update his behavior a bit.

At the risk of appearing to blame the victim, it is nevertheless true that women are often ambivalent about their own roles. On the one hand, we want to end the discussions and get on with life, free of the domestic demands that are so draining and exhausting. On the other hand, we have traditionally been conditioned to nurture and to serve, and deep inside we fear that if we renounce that traditional role and refute "the need to be needed," we will risk losing part of our feminine identity. And then there are the men and the children we love. In the ultimate irony of ironies, even a self-proclaimed feminist will often rationalize her husband's uncooperative behavior and sacrifice her own values and beliefs to preserve her marriage.

The solution for the previous generation of women caught in this gender gap was the creation of superwoman/supermom, the woman who could do it all and walk on water in her spare time. But, as one family therapist so aptly put it, "The problem with the superwoman/supermom is that she robs everyone else in the family of their competence, and then blames them for letting her do it." Need we say any more about female ambivalence?

From Past to Present

Marital roles and expectations are shaped mainly by our childhood experiences and a conscious effort to repeat, or not repeat, what our parents did. So, if you had a stay-at-home mom and found that comforting, you would probably like to stay home with your own children one day. Is it realistic to hope that you'll be able to afford to do that? Will you have to sacrifice career advancement forever if you do? Or, maybe you had an executive mom, whom you admired and hoped to emulate, but now that you find yourself on the fast track, you're positively breathless already. Can you imagine adding motherhood to this mix? How did she do it all? Did she do it as effortlessly as you remember?

There are no easy answers, and the choice is not always yours alone. Even if you and your husband can come to some agreement about domestic divisions and marital roles, there are still influences in society that directly affect your decisions, factors such as the economy, available child care, flexible work hours, and parental leave.

So, here we are, back to precedents again, because sorting the laundry and cleaning the vegetables may seem inconsequential right now, but your decisions about who does what can have long-term implications. If you readily accept "the second shift," as the best-selling book by the same name dubbed it, you'll almost certainly come to resent your situation, especially when the house gets bigger, the career gets more demanding, and the kids come along. And, if you divide the labor in your home on a gender-role basis, then what other rights, roles, and responsibilities will also be divided on the basis of sex? Think about it.

Conflict over domestic duties is second only to money as a constant source of marital discord (and, often, the two issues are related). Maybe that's because the division of household labor, more than any other single issue, is perceived by most women as an indicator of fairness and equity in marriage. And, as at least one important study of newlywed satisfaction has shown, perceptions of fairness and equity are directly related to feelings of marital well-being (Blair & Johnson).

Household Solutions

So, what can you do about all this? How can you find reasonable, commonsense solutions to life's everyday demands that you can both live with? Here are some answers that have worked for other couples.

Buy whatever help you need.
This includes not only household cleaning help on a weekly or biweekly basis, but also professional cleaning services that come in periodically for heavy-duty jobs. You can also take those shirts to the professional laundry, get a lawn ser-

---

What Other Couples Say . . .

A National Survey of Families and Households, conducted among both cohabiting and married couples in 1988, found that women performed an average of 33 hours of housework per week, not including child care, compared to men's average of 14 hours per week.

By the way, in another study, wives admitted to making the bed 96 percent of the time, but husbands do 86 percent of all household repairs (Blair & Johnson, 570-71).

---

vice to cut the grass and trim the shrubbery, pay a neighborhood teenager to do seasonal chores (raking leaves, washing windows, etc.), buy take-out meals, and even use professional shopping services to save time and energy (for your wardrobe, interior decorating, holiday gifts, etc.). Of course, the main ingredient here is money, but buying auxiliary services has proven to be the answer for many, many couples, even those on relatively tight budgets.

"I was the only one working and James was in school," says Paula, "so we didn't have that much money. But even then I had a cleaning woman come in every other week. It was worth it to me. My mother always had help, so to me it's just basic. It's not a luxury, it's a necessity."

Divide chores by whoever is in the best position
to do them most efficiently.

Forget gender roles as a basis for division; use common sense. Who's up last in the morning? That person should make the bed. Who's home first in the evening? That person should start dinner. Can the last one to leave in the morning throw in a load of laundry, and the first one home transfer it to the dryer? Can one of you run the vacuum while the other scrubs the bathroom in the evening? Somehow, chores done together, or simultaneously, seem less a burden than those done alone.

The idea here is not to divide the list by a rigid formula, but for each of you to pitch in to get routine tasks incorporated into your weekday schedules. That way repetitive chores get taken care of during the week, and you two have your weekend relatively free to do fun things together.

Honor skills and preferences whenever possible.

Again, forget gender stereotypes; who wants to do what? You may find this hard to believe, but some people actually *do* like to cook, or iron, or fold laundry, or weed flower beds. And some people actually hate to grocery shop, or sort and pay bills, or mow the grass. As much as possible, then, try to allocate your chores by personal preference. With a little luck, maybe neither of you will have to do something you absolutely hate, at least not all the time.

"My husband really loves to cook, and plan meals, and grocery shop," Sandy says, "so I figure great! Me? I find opening a can of soup stressful, so his taking complete charge of food is worth a lifetime of my doing the laundry." Sounds like a fair trade, doesn't it?

Evaluate the necessity of some chores.

Just because your mother soaked the venetian blinds in the bathtub, does that mean you have to? People used to beat rugs and scrub woodwork regularly, too. Some chores are more of a habit or a ritual than an actual necessity, so you really need to rethink their importance in light of all the other demands on your time.

Also, look for ways to streamline the chores you do have to do. For instance, must the furniture be dusted with a cloth and polish, or will a quick swish with a feather duster do? One tip: if you keep household clutter to a minimum and both try to pick up after yourselves at the end of each day, your home will always appear cleaner than it is.

Consider maintenance before you buy.

That glass-topped coffee table may look great in the showroom, but how will it look with the sun streaming over its dusty top in your living room? Ornate furniture with intricate details to dust; silver, copper, and brass that have to be polished; solid wood floors that have to be waxed and buffed—all these may be accoutrements of the good life, but only if you have a staff to take care of them.

The same considerations apply to larger purchases, too, such as moving to a bigger apartment or buying a house. "I never would have believed the difference going from a condo to a house could make," says Larry, a newlywed homeowner. "It's not only the money, all the repairs and renovations and unexpected expenses that come up, but it's also the time. Seems like Linda and I spend every spare minute we have working around the house because, inside and out, there is *always* something that has to be done." Ah, yes, the joys of homeownership!

Appreciate each other.

Regrettably, the people we love most are the ones we're most likely to take for granted. Don't be stingy with the "pleases" and "thank-yous" or neglect to pay a compliment for a job well done. For that matter, even if the job isn't so well done, or isn't done exactly the way you would do it, be grateful. After all, who cares whether all the towels are facing in the same direction in the linen closet? The important thing is that they made it there!

One of the terrible realities of modern life is that everybody tries to do so much. You come home in the evening after a long day and face cooking, cleaning, laundry, paperwork—it seems never-ending, especially when you're tired and irritable. It's easy to start bickering over the housework, over who did what when or whose turn it is now, because neither of you really wants to deal with any of it.

A good way to avoid this kind of petty nagging and nitpicking is by a general agreement, arrived at when you're both calm and rested, on who is responsible for what so you don't have to renegotiate the same tasks all the time. Truthfully, better that some chores don't get done at all than the two of you get undone trying to do them.

Problems of Relocation

Of all the difficult adjustments every newlywed couple has to face, perhaps none is more difficult than the relocation of one of the partners to a strange new locale right after the wedding. Moving is stressful anytime, but especially so when you combine it with another major life change.

To begin with, the relocated spouse may know next to nothing about the physical layout of the area. Finding stores, churches, theaters, or restaurants, even the way back to one's own home, can become a major challenge, to say nothing of job hunting or learning to navigate public transportation in a big city. It's unnerving to have to rely on maps and schedules for your every move.

And then there's the matter of services: doctors, dentists, hairdressers/barbers, grocery stores, drugstores, dry cleaners, banks. . . . The newcomer could ask somebody for recommendations if he or she knew anyone or had any friends to ask. And that's another story.

What all this boils down to is tremendous pressure on the nonrelocated spouse to try to smooth the way, give directions, make introductions, find out, explain, support, and encourage. And, until the newcomer has friends and colleagues of his or her own, the hometown spouse will also have to provide the only relief from loneliness.

Cross-country or international moves are particularly difficult because the culture and the way of life, maybe even the language, will be different and will take some getting used to. Also, a move of great distance usually means that old friends and family have been left behind, so an old-fashioned case of homesickness is to be expected. Nor does an "instant family" of new relatives and friends make the transition any easier; often, it's just the opposite. The newcomer feels obligated to like and accept these people, and that, in turn, creates pressures and resentments of a different sort. (See more about integration of family and friends in Chapter 4.)

If one of you has relocated for the sake of the other, you will both have to be patient until you have both settled in. Here are some tips that might ease the transition:

- Employment is the quickest, easiest way to get immersed in a new community. Even if an early offer isn't the job of your dreams, take it just to have something and to get acclimated. You can always find a better job later.
- Churches/synagogues provide good ways to meet people. Most religious congregations welcome newcomers and offer myriad opportunities for service and social activities.

- Don't wait for the neighbors in your apartment complex or on your street to come greet you; go introduce yourself to them. They will be good sources of information on local services and resources—and complaints. Besides, you should know who your neighbors are.
- If you were active in a national club or organization where you lived before, see if there's a local chapter you might join.
- If you've relocated to a foreign country, take language lessons. You will never feel at home until you can speak the language.
- Go out and explore, map in hand. You can only learn a place by actually navigating it. If you get lost, you'll eventually find your way back, and then you'll know a lot more about the territory than you did when you set out.

Personal Resources Worksheet

Doctors

General:
Address: Phone:

OB/GYN:
Address: Phone:

Specialist:
Address: Phone:

Dentist:
Address: Phone:

Ophthalmologist:
Address: Phone:

Veterinarian:
Address: Phone:

Pharmacist:
Address: Phone:

Advisors

Attorney:
Address: Phone:

Accountant:
Address: Phone:

Banker/Broker:
Address: Phone:

Financial Planner:
Address: Phone:

Clergy:
Address: Phone:

Diet/Fitness:
Address: Phone:

Travel Agent:
Address: Phone:

Insurance Contacts

Agency:
Address: Phone:

Auto:
Address: Phone:

Homeowners:
Address: Phone:

Life:
Address: Phone:

Health/Disability:
Address: Phone:

Household Services

Plumber:
Address: Phone:

Electrician:
Address: Phone:

Heating/Air Conditioning:
Address: Phone:

Security System:
Address: Phone:

Housekeeper:
Address: Phone:

Handyman:
Address: Phone:

Gardener:
Address: Phone:

Newspaper Service:
Address: Phone:

Hairdresser:
Address: Phone:

Auto Mechanic:
Address: Phone:

Other

CHAPTER 2

Establishing Your Couplehood

*A*t first, he was another new man in your life, and you were the new woman in his. You flirted, you courted, you played coquettish games. Then you got to know each other better and, gradually, the two of you became "an item." And then you realized you were really in love, and love turned into commitment.

"Going into business for yourself is both scary and exciting," says George, an accountant who recently opened his own small firm. "You have to be honest with yourself about your assets and liabilities, you have to be absolutely determined to make it, and you have to keep your sense of humor and try not to take every little thing *too* seriously." The same could be said for the business of marriage and, since George is also a newlywed, he can use his own advice. Marriage is a major career move, one that demands all the energy, planning, and dedication that any new venture requires. The work doesn't end when you say "I do," any more than it does your first day on the job. The two of you are a couple now, a true partnership in every sense of the word, and this is only the beginning.

Me Vs. We

Your decision to marry reflects an awareness of your need for another significant person in your life and an acceptance of the interdependency such a need creates. But, the challenge of balancing your personal goals and needs with those of your mate will present an ongoing challenge to your self-esteem and identity. Who should do what? What's most important? Whose needs come first? Where do "we" end and "I" begin? Those aren't easy questions, and out of your answers will evolve your marital roles.

"I thought I understood Mark's dedication to his career," says Helen, three years of marriage and one child later, "because I have similar career ambitions. But, now that the baby's come, I feel like I'm the only one making concessions and pushing myself to fill all the roles: professional person, parent, and spouse. Mark has made virtually no adjustments at all. He still works late, travels a lot, and

---

❧❧❧ DO YOU SEE YOURSELF HERE? ❧❧❧

- Do you feel some loss of independence since the marriage, some inconvenience at having to worry about another person?
- Are you still having marital adjustments even if you and your spouse lived together before marriage?
- Are you having difficulties settling into comfortable marital roles?
- Are you surprised at how difficult it is to really talk and really listen to each other about very important things?
- Do you argue more than you thought you would?
- Do you sometimes feel guilty because you feel crowded or need more privacy?
- Do you feel a need for a spiritual center; have you abandoned practicing your religious faith since marriage?
- Are you facing a crisis in your lives right now that is straining the marriage?
- Are you surprised at the kind of couple you're turning out to be?

A number of "yes" answers? Read on.

---

expects everything at home to take care of itself. We made the decision to have a child together, so why am I the only one feeling pressured and compromised?"

Why indeed? Perhaps Helen feels compromised (and maybe Mark does, too, even though he isn't showing it) because it's relatively easy to be sure of who you are and what you want when you're unencumbered—single. You can set your own priorities and make the choices that are in your best interest. But once you're married, the needs and desires of your spouse and family members become intrinsic to the harmony and happiness in your own life. When too many priorities present themselves at once, you feel overwhelmed, even resentful as Helen does, because the burden of choice is upon you. That is when you find yourself asking where the "we" ends and the "I" begins.

The pull between independence and togetherness is especially hard for today's couples, who have probably been more focused on their individual educational and career goals, and who are older and therefore more accustomed to being single. Society's emphasis on self-sufficiency and competition does not reconcile easily to the kind of interdependency and cooperation demanded in marriage. Having to consider another in every decision you make, personal and professional, poses one of the more difficult transitions from the single to the married lifestyle.

No matter how well you think you know yourself, marriage will require a new level of maturity and an increased sense of selflessness and of self. And, no matter how well you think you know each other before marriage, you will be surprised at how differently you perceive the actions of your spouse once you are legally bound. Nothing quite prepares you for the magnitude of those changes.

Life after Marriage

The change in attitudes and perceptions after marriage comes as a real shock to couples who have been living together before, because conventional wisdom has it that living together allows two people a realistic preview of what their married life will be like. Well, maybe . . . or maybe not.

"Look, I was engaged once before and it fell apart," says Steve, "because she wanted to change who I was and what I did. I finally figured out that she didn't want to live the life I had to offer, but it was hurtful to learn that so late in the game."

Steve is the quintessential entrepreneur. An admitted workaholic who loves what he does and spends 60 to 70 hours a week doing it, he can already claim significant professional and financial success at age 32. His life is exciting and fast paced but, of course, there is a downside.

"I travel a great deal, do a lot of business entertaining, and am on the phone, fax, or computer constantly when I'm home. That's not easy to live with, I know," he admits. "So, when I met Carol and we decided we were in love, I wanted her to know exactly what kind of a life she was getting into. That's why we decided to live together before we got married, to be sure we could both handle the realities of this situation."

They could and they did, and Steve and Carol are a married couple now. Their cohabitation, which lasted one year and during which time they also planned their wedding, was consciously intended to be a period of preparation for the marriage. But not all couples live together first for such concrete reasons and for such a finite amount of time.

Estimates are that today almost half of all American marriages are preceded by a preliminary period of living together that lasts anywhere from a few months to several years. Contrary to popular belief, though, longer periods of cohabitation do not necessarily result in easier transitions into marriage and more stable, lasting relationships. In fact, recent studies in Canada, Sweden, and the United States have proven the opposite to be true (Thomson & Colella, 259). The probability for future success and happiness, however, may have more to do with the reasons couples lived together than with the fact that they did (Schoen, 281).

If you and your spouse lived together before marriage because you weren't sure of the relationship or because one of you couldn't make a commitment, then chances are you've had still more difficult adjustments to make after the marriage. That's because the ground rules for marriage are very different from the ground rules in a purely romantic, "maybe this will work" relationship. During a trial period, even one that goes on for years, partners persist in certain courtship behaviors: they maintain some individual autonomy and independence; they avoid conflict and let many issues slide; they are generally not intimately involved with each other's families; and they don't discuss marital roles because marriage is not yet a certainty. The future is viewed as an "if," not a "when," and decisions are pretty much day-to-day.

Even though the routines of everyday life don't change that much after marriage, the perception of the relationship and of each partner's role in it changes dramatically for such couples. The permanence of it all, the loss of singlehood forever, the shared responsibilities for families and friends, the long-term decision making, and the new awareness of the other as integral to one's own fate—all this brings new meaning, and immediacy, to the roles of husband and wife.

Ironically, family therapists note that couples who have had stormy relationships during cohabitation, or those who have actually sought premarital counseling, find the transition into marriage easier and the resulting union more stable. Maybe that's because, like Steve and Carol, they never doubted the seriousness of their commitment to each other, and so have used the period of living together to begin the work of resolving the problems and issues between them.

Marital Roles

Men provide, women nurture. Do you agree? What happens when circumstances dictate otherwise? What happens when roles are reversed?

When we think of marital roles, most of us automatically think in terms of gender roles and marriage models, particularly traditional ones like Ozzie and Harriet. But, there's a great deal more involved in the delineation of marital roles than just who does the housework or who brings home the bacon. Rather, these assigned and assumed roles become the permanent part we play in the larger relationship, one through which, ideally, each partner's physical and emotional needs are met and each is enabled to thrive and grow.

For the most part, we tend to replicate what we witnessed as children in our parents' relationship, even when we don't want to. "Paul and I both come from extremely similar, fairly traditional, intact families in which the fathers are successful career men, but passive and deferential at home, and the mothers are the dominant decision makers and much more emotionally expressive and assertive," says Cheryl. "Both of us have had some difficulty standing up to our mothers, and so both of us agreed before marriage that ours would be a more

---

What Other Couples Say . . .

Newlywed husbands are likely to report that their spouses are the overbenefited partners in marriage and that they are the underbenefited. Newlywed women tend to agree. Researchers conclude that, at least at the early stages of marriage, males consider themselves trapped (Crohan & Veroff, 387).

Is this the typical story of the male's mythic loss of freedom, or is it that today's husbands finally realize that they're going to have to give, as well as get, at home?

mutually expressive, shared-decision-making kind of relationship. I've made a conscious effort to temper my take-charge attitude and my outspoken reactions to situations, and Paul has tried to be more open and honest in expressing his ideas and opinions, and more involved in the domestic aspects of our life, like home furnishings and family affairs."

The result? Almost all the couple's arguments stem from their struggle with marital roles. (Remember their honeymoon tiff?) "In spite of ourselves," Cheryl marvels, "I still turn into my mother, and his, and Paul still turns into his father, and mine. I get insistent, he becomes withdrawn, and we both see it, but we can't stop it. This role thing is turning into the biggest challenge of our marriage."

The "role thing" is every couple's biggest challenge; the difference is that Paul and Cheryl are smart enough to know it. Their ongoing struggle shows how strong family patterns are and how difficult it is to unlearn the behaviors learned in childhood. Either you inadvertently become the child you were again in your adult relationship, or you find yourself behaving toward your spouse the way your parents behaved toward you.

Dr. Harville Hendrix, well-known marital therapist and author of *Getting the Love You Want* and *Keeping the Love You Find,* has helped millions better understand the repetition of old family dramas in their lives and what that means to their present relationships. "Whatever happens in childhood, whether it's mild or intense, there is something that's going to replicate itself in adulthood in an intimate partnership," says Dr. Hendrix. "And it always has to be repaired in a relationship in adulthood with somebody similar to your parents."

The only way to alter such patterns is to become aware of them and then to make a conscious decision to act in different ways. But, both of you have to learn to recognize what these patterns are, and both of you have to agree to change them.

In Cheryl and Paul's case, it's not so much that their parents' marital role model is destructive as that it is outdated (the silent male and the emotive female). Modern couples don't want to accept the old gender stereotypes, and most don't want the kind of marriage models such stereotypes produce. Instead, they want a more equitable partnership in which both spouses give and get, at home and at work, and both participate more fully in the emotional life of the family. At least, that's what women seem to expect. But, as discussed in a *Glamour* magazine article, many experts feel that men are lagging behind, still secretly longing to give at work and get at home (Tenlin, 266).

Being fully participational does not mean that both partners give and get in equal measure in every situation, however, but both have to care about each other and the relationship. Equality is found in the overall balance of needs met and care given, and the subtle shifts in dominance between partners from one situation to the next. The idea is that no one spouse be completely dominant in the relationship and have virtually all needs met, while the other does all the giving and all the giving in.

It's hard to strike that balance. Both spouses have to be very sure of who they are and what they're about, and not everyone has that level of maturity and self-confidence in early marriage. And then there are those who cling to tradi-

Six Marriage Models

Do you see your parents' model here, or that of other couples you know? How well do their marriages work? Which model seems to be evolving for the two of you?

Type	*Characteristics*	*Comments*
Tarzan and Jane	Male completely dominant, maybe even abusive, in all things; woman totally dependent and subservient, treated as chattel.	Doesn't even belong in the jungle!
Daddy Bear/ Mommy Bear	Male dominant, although perhaps as a benevolent dictator; female is full-time homemaker and is dependent on him for status and support.	A nineteenth-century model that has left a lot of women high and dry in twentieth-century divorce courts.
Power behind the Throne	Traditional roles of male as primary breadwinner and female as primary caretaker make it appear as though he is head of household, but he is only the titular head; hers is the real power to move and manipulate.	1950's nostalgia dies hard.
Role Reversal	The woman as primary provider and the man as primary caretaker, maybe even househusband.	An increasingly common corollary to the rise of entrepreneurship and working at home.
The Corporation	Both partners are competent and accomplished, and each has special "spheres of influence," but one (usually the man) is likely to make more money and, therefore, to enjoy slightly more status and autonomy.	A common late twentieth-century model, probably due to the pro-liferation of MBA degrees.
The True Partnership	Husband and wife share equal responsibility for everything, and their roles are interchangeable and without gender bias. All decision making is joint.	An ideal, but still seldom a living reality.

tional roles: the men who won't change a diaper or the women who won't change a tire because the stereotypes are all they know, regardless of how inconvenient and unworkable those stereotypes are in meeting the demands of contemporary life.

The two of you are probably working through some of these issues right now, just as countless other newlywed couples are. That work will continue for a long time because marital roles evolve, slowly. They even change slightly over time as situations change. What doesn't change, however, are the valuable negotiating strategies and communication skills you develop as you wrestle to determine who you are as people and what kind of couple you want to be.

Effective Communication

Americans are the most information/communication conscious people in the world. Why, then, do we find communicating with those we love so difficult? Or is it that we expect our loved ones to read our minds?

"What's wrong, dear?"

"Nothing."

Right.

Communication is about letting the other person in, not just when there's a problem or conflict, but all the time. It's about exchanging ideas, sharing burdens, solving problems, and bolstering each other's confidence and self-esteem. Most of all, it's about being actively engaged with each other, paying attention not only to the literal messages, but to the wants, needs, fears, and desires underneath.

While we commonly think of communication as a dialogue, an oral exchange, remember that there are all sorts of other ways to communicate: body language, laughter, facial expression and eye contact, touch, sex, written messages, personal favors, gifts and surprises, even silence. We tend to forget about these nonverbal techniques, many of which we used quite effectively during courtship. They can be just as effective now and for the rest of your life, maybe even more effective as you get to know each other better.

In marriage, it is vitally important that each of you learn to respect what the other thinks and feels, and that you develop reliable methods for exchanging those thoughts and feelings for mutual understanding. You may not face the monumental decisions typical of longer-married couples right away, but the patterns of relating and the skills you employ in communicating about small, everyday issues will be the same patterns and skills you'll bring to bigger, more important discussions later on. That's why you need to develop strategies that work.

Learning to express yourself in a clear and appropriate way and learning to be an active listener takes time and practice. You have to discover ways to relate to each other that work for you, and they may not necessarily be the same ways your families or your friends communicate. In addition, married couples can't afford a long list of subjects that are taboo as topics of conversation. You have to be able to talk about anything that's important to you, including sex, money, religion, politics, or in-laws. Otherwise, you risk alienation and withdrawal, and you create a climate in which communication about anything becomes strained.

Programs such as Marriage Encounter and Marriage Enrichment focus on developing couple communication skills through dialogue. In workshops and weekend retreats, couples explore the ways they relate to each other and affirm their commitment to their marriages. One such marriage enrichment agency is The Association for Couples in Marriage Enrichment (A.C.M.E.). "A.C.M.E. is not an organization of therapists and these are not therapy sessions," emphasizes Susan deGuzman, Director of Communications. "Our motto is: making good marriages better, beginning with our own." A.C.M.E. is unique in that skills are learned through couple and group exercises and sharing sessions in a variety of settings. (See Appendix for resource.)

Following are some of the communication strategies that A.C.M.E. teaches:

1. Set aside time every day to talk. It doesn't matter whether you talk about the little things or the big things in your lives, just as long as you talk.
2. Confront petty annoyances on a daily basis, preferably, if possible, when they arise. Getting annoyed with your partner is natural. You have a better chance of handling annoyances with each other in a positive way if you do so before they become too numerous and blown out of proportion. If all you can do at times is admit anger, this in itself will be helpful.
3. Explain, don't complain. Use "I" sentences ("I feel hurt when . . . ") rather than accusing "you" sentences ("You made me angry when you . . . ") that put your partner on the defensive.
4. Be a good listener. Listen with your eyes and your ears. "Body talk" (demeanor, subtle gestures, facial expression, tone of voice, etc.) is very telling.
5. Use feedback and clarification to ensure that you fully understand what your partner is saying to avoid complicating issues with misunderstandings.
6. Be available and approachable. Try not to be so preoccupied with other concerns that you can't be interested in the issues at hand.
7. Be patient and use a warm, friendly tone of voice. Politeness is basic to all human relations.
8. Give your partner the space he or she needs. Ask for space when you need it, too. Encourage communication, but don't force information. Allow your partner to have his or her own private thoughts and feelings. Trust that communication about a particular issue will come at a better time.
9. Be aware of what's going on inside of yourself—what you are feeling, thinking, wanting, doing, etc. Without an awareness of the impact of daily pressures, partners may tend to blame each other for the irritations they are feeling.
10. Put yourself in your partner's shoes and try to understand how he or she experiences life.

Creative Conflict

When communication breaks down, conflict ensues, right? Well, not necessarily. Communication makes it possible to work through conflict, which is inevitable between two people, and to come out whole on the other side.

"We had to agree to disagree," Harold says flatly about his wife's decision to accept a teaching fellowship at a university rather than a more financially feasible position in industry. "I gave in," he continues, "because this fellowship seemed to be an unusual opportunity for Lynette and because, in fairness, it *was* her decision to make. I'm still concerned about our finances, but I guess it will all work out."

Lynette's freedom of choice in this decision was complicated by increased expenses due to the couple's recent purchase of their first home and Harold's growing dissatisfaction with his present career track. In fact, it had been her initial suggestion a few months ago that they both look for "more gainful employment" as a step toward a more secure financial future. Ironically, just as she was about to accept a higher-paying position, the offer of a university fellowship came her way.

"There are some long-term advantages to a career in academia," Lynette points out. "I'll be furthering my formal education while broadening my work experience. And, since we'd like to have a family one day, I feel the flexibility of a teaching/research schedule is important."

Harold and Lynette wrestled with this decision, even argued about it, for weeks because, basically, they could not reconcile two entirely different points of view: he tends to worry more about money and to equate job worth with earning power, while she generally has a more relaxed attitude about money and approaches career choices with an eye toward more than financial gains. Neither viewpoint is wrong, and in fact, Harold and Lynette usually count on their differing attitudes to bring balance to their partnership. But this time, the balance wasn't easy to strike.

"Once I got over feeling guilty about not making an equal financial contribution to our marriage, and once Harold admitted that he would probably worry about money no matter what our income was, I was freed to make a decision that felt right for me," Lynette says. "But it took us a long time to get down to the real issues in this discussion, and each of us had to give a little. Harold had to defer to my right to make a career decision based on what would be more satisfying and less stressful for me, and in return, I have agreed to pick up more of the slack at home so he can devote more energy to his more high-powered career goals."

Compromise, concessions, negotiations. It sounds like a business deal—and it is. Ultimately, when you can't agree wholeheartedly, someone gives in because no one person's needs and opinions should have automatic priority all the time. The real creativity in conflict is found in the way trade-offs are made; even if both partners don't come away from the situation feeling that they have both won, at least neither has to walk away feeling he or she has suffered an undue loss.

"The Four Horsemen of the Apocalypse"

Seattle psychologist Dr. John Gottman at the University of Washington has been studying couples' interaction styles, particularly how they perform tasks and react to conflict. By videotaping their behaviors, he has been able to analyze body language and facial expressions, as well as verbal exchanges, and to identify four key behaviors that he believes are truly "apocalyptic" for the marriage:

1. Criticism
2. Defensiveness
3. Contempt
4. Withdrawal from interaction

"It's interesting," Lynette adds as a footnote. "When we told my parents our news, their initial reactions mirrored our own. Mother thought I was making a wise choice, while Dad wondered whether I could really afford to do what I wanted to do at this particular time. And it was Harold who came to the defense of my decision, explaining in detail how this choice made more sense for both of us in the long run!"

The return to a unified front after a conflict has been resolved is not only a sign of successful negotiation strategies, but it is also the only positive way to get past whatever conflict existed. It's important to distinguish between disagreements and all-out arguments. Two people can disagree about lots of things, but still coexist peacefully and happily—"agree to disagree," as Harold put it. Arguments, on the other hand, usually erupt because someone loses emotional control and then says or does something that is hurtful and inflames the situation. When voices rise, reason departs.

Arguments are normal and every couple has them; after all, if you didn't care, you wouldn't argue. (Apathy, not hatred, is the true opposite of love.) It is not the number of arguments you have, nor even what you argue about that poses danger to the relationship. Rather, it's the way the arguments are conducted and the way you each feel after they're over. When you seriously hurt each other, you seriously hurt the marriage.

Learn to fight fair, to forgive, and to say "I'm sorry." Lingering regrets and recriminations are the death knell to a healthy relationship. Don't let them sound in your head; voice them, settle them one way or another, and move on.

Privacy and Respect

Certainly, talking and sharing, and even creative conflict, build stronger communication skills, and solid communication is a foundation for a stronger marriage. But here's a viewpoint on the virtues of silence that's worth considering, from someone who's been married for 35 years:

"Some subjects are better not approached, and some questions are better not asked. I know the tendency today is for everyone to talk everything to death, but we all have private places in ourselves. When you love someone, you learn to recognize, and to respect, those private places—and to leave them alone."

Privacy. It's a word we don't hear too often in our talk-show, tabloid world, but it's an important concept, and a fundamental right, even in marriage. Sometimes, in lovers' overzealous efforts to know and understand everything about each other, the natural needs for privacy get misinterpreted and the rights to privacy get trampled.

Do You Fight Fair?

Take this quiz to see if you fight fair, or if you need to work on this area. Answer yes or no to each of the following questions, then tally your score and compare your answers.

1. Do you "speak up" when something really bothers you, rather than suppressing your anger for days until you're ready to explode?
2. Can you control your temper when the time or place is inappropriate for an emotional outburst?
3. Do you argue in private without an audience of friends or relatives?
4. Do you look beyond the incident that triggered your anger to the real source of misunderstanding?
5. Do you keep the discussion to the issue at hand rather than dragging in old hurts and past wrongs?
6. Do you listen during an argument and honestly try to hear the other person's point of view?
7. Do you avoid the accusatory "you" and concentrate on the "I-we" instead?
8. Do you refrain from making idle threats and delivering ultimatums?
9. Do you have the ability to say "I'm sorry" or "I was wrong"?
10. Can you hold your ground and not just "give in" when you feel your position justified?
11. Do you seek a firm resolution to each conflict so arguments don't compound themselves?
12. Are you willing to compromise when a clear-cut resolution doesn't seem to present itself?
13. Do you "get over" the disagreement once it's resolved rather than pouting and sulking for days?
14. Can you leave the irritations of your day at the office and not take them out on your spouse?
15. Can you remember that not every minor infraction is worth arguing over?

Total the number of "yes" answers: 15—Congratulations! You're a lover, not a fighter. 10–14—At least you're fair. Below 10—Remember: never go to bed angry.

"I think we just need more space, literally and figuratively," says Beverly about the constant bickering and arguing that go on between her and her husband. When the couple married, they moved into his small studio apartment for what they thought would be only a month or two until they found something bigger. But, a lost job and a tight economy have kept them in the small apartment for over a year.

"We're on top of each other. My papers and schoolwork get all mixed up with his resumes and letters and phone messages. In a one-room studio, the only place either of us can be alone is in the bathroom," Beverly says. "It's given us cabin fever; we just can't get away from each other."

The space crunch is especially hard for this couple because they each had lived alone for several years before the marriage, and they each have professions (she's a teacher, he's an architect) that require a good deal of at-home work. So, Beverly is convinced, probably correctly, that the cramped physical space has created concurrent feelings of being emotionally cramped as well. With their physical freedom restricted, and their personal and professional privacy invaded, both have grown unusually irritable.

Togetherness should not be confused with emotional closeness; in fact, too much togetherness can actually stifle closeness (which is probably where the "absence makes the heart grow fonder" adage came from). People need their own space. If one of you works at home or is involved in hobbies or crafts, you will need proportionately more space to accommodate those activities. If you are lucky enough to have a home with several rooms, you'll soon find that each of you naturally starts to claim certain spots in the house, to read, or work, or just sit. You need privacy for phone calls, private places to sit and chat with friends, places to be alone and think, and neither of you should feel threatened by those needs in the other.

If you don't have the luxury of all the space you need, try these tactics for expanding what you do have into places of your own:

- If you live in a small apartment, you will have to settle for less personal space, but you can still stake out drawers, desks, or tabletops, and favorite chairs or spots on the couch.
- A personal space, once claimed, should not be violated. If your parents ever read your diary or snooped around in your room, then you know what violation means. If you have a desk drawer, you have the right to expect that your partner won't go rifling through it for no reason. If one of you gets a letter in the mail, the other shouldn't open it. Respect means trusting each other and resisting the temptation to intrude.
- It's okay to want to be alone sometimes. Try taking a walk or going to the health club regularly for a workout. The two of you may have merged into one couple, but you're still two individuals, and a desire for solitude is not unnatural.
- Married or not, each of you is still your own person. You are entitled to have your own friends, your own conversations, and your own confidences without necessarily including your spouse. Neither of you should feel resentful or left out when the other exercises that right.

- You are also entitled to your own opinions, which you may or may not choose to express. You two will not always agree, but you should both always feel comfortable saying what you think.

One of the truly ongoing joys of married life is the continual unfolding of the mysteries of the other, the small, slow revelations of the complexities of personality and character in your spouse that cause your love to deepen and grow. Paradoxically, only a genuine respect for the privacy of each individual will allow those revelations to occur.

Shared Spiritual Values

What do you believe in? Is there someone, or something, greater than yourself? Are you one of the 92 percent of all Americans who, according to The National Study of Religious Identification, profess some religious affiliation? Is that profession of faith a part of your lives as a couple?

Study after study, from national polls to independent research, has shown positive correlations between a couple's religious values and their marital happiness. And, an overwhelming majority of weddings are religious ceremonies. So why don't more couples give more attention to the discussion and development of a shared spirituality?

"I think religion is like sex and money," says Jody, 32. "People are uncomfortable discussing it."

Jody and her husband, Augie, are Roman Catholic, and both are active in their parish. She is a special minister, he sings in the choir, and each of them teaches in the youth religious education program. "I don't think of us as being super Catholics or anything, but our friends tease us for being soooo religious just because we go to church every Sunday," Jody says. "At first, the teasing bothered me, but over time, as I've watched how other couples deal with things, or fail to, I feel that Augie and I have a cohesion and a direction that they don't have. Our faith seems to enable us to take the knocks of life better."

Among religious and lay experts alike, that seems to be the consensus: a shared spirituality provides a sense of values and purpose in life and a common source of strength. It doesn't matter what a couple believes, as long as they believe in something greater than themselves. It doesn't even seem to matter so much if the partners have different religions, as long as they can emphasize the positive and share a common moral and spiritual core.

Having the same religion has obvious benefits, of course, in that both spouses will see their marriage the same way—as an indissoluble sacrament, for instance, or as a metaphor for the covenant between God and His people. The same holiday traditions and religious rituals can be enjoyed by all family members, and the question of how to raise the children will never come up. However, sharing the same faith doesn't always mean you practice it the same way.

Jody again: "Believe it or not, Augie and I have argued a lot about religion in these first years of our marriage because he and I were raised as different types of Roman Catholics. My family is ethnic Catholic, dogmatic and religious in a symbolic, but very personal way. We had crucifixes in every room and a novena for every cause. My mother even buried a statue of St. Joseph in the ground once when she wanted to sell the house.

"Augie's family is less emotional, more practical about their religion. They go to church because it is an important part of their lives, but they didn't discuss their Catholic philosophy and beliefs, and they don't interpret all the rules and regulations literally. So, what I discovered was that while Augie and I professed belief in the same religion, in some ways, we visualized a different God."

The Challenge for Interfaith Couples

Jody and Augie have worked out their interpretational differences by both moving a bit toward center and by making distinctions between common religious beliefs and differing ethical stands on some contemporary issues. They've discovered that spiritual values and beliefs can be intensely personal and emotional, and that no amount of discussion or debate can dislodge deeply held convictions.

However complicated discussions of spirituality can become for couples of the same faith, interfaith couples have even more of a challenge, and often their families and religious communities offer nothing but indifference or downright hostility. "In spite of our growing numbers, interfaith families have a difficult time finding information and help," says Joan Hawxhurst, editor and founder of *Dovetail,* a Jewish–Christian newsletter. "These couples often end up angry and alienated, and that's not good for them or the marriage." Hawxhurst founded her publication to help.

Ongoing surveys by the Council of Jewish Federations show that approximately 52 percent of all Jewish men and women take gentile spouses, and the National Opinion Research Center at the University of Chicago estimates that over a third of all Roman Catholics are involved in what are called "mixed marriages." There are no reliable figures for other types of intermarriage among other Christian sects and between Christians and non-Christians, but we do know a basic fact: regardless of how families and theologians feel about it, the religious and cultural identities of Americans are undergoing dramatic transformations. And that means so will the traditions, rituals, and religious values of these newly amalgamated couples. (See Chapter 4 for more on interfaith marriage.)

Don't abandon the goal of nourishing the spiritual center in your lives just because you are an interfaith couple. Search for one of the growing number of interfaith support groups through which the two of you can discuss religious issues with other interfaith couples, and try to find a faith community that will welcome you both. You can explore other religions to see if a third compromise would be acceptable, or you might each continue to practice your respective faiths alone, integrating both religious traditions at home.

Most of all, respect each other's heritage and persevere. Look to the God who brought you together and count yourselves lucky that you have twice as much faith to live by, rather than no faith at all. (See the Appendix for interfaith resources, and Chapters 3 and 4 for more on religious and cultural issues among families.)

Interfaith or not, if you have been lackadaisical about your spiritual life before marriage, maybe it's time now to explore the satisfactions and support a religion can offer. Visit some congregations in your area and try to find one that makes you both feel welcome. You might also try making some religious observance part of major holiday celebrations and special occasions during the year. Even something as simple as a prayer of thanksgiving before meals reinforces a habit of shared faith and religious values. Statistics prove it: the couple who prays together, stays together (Greeley, 190).

Customs and Traditions

As newlyweds, you each bring a host of cultural, religious, and family traditions to marriage. The more disparate your backgrounds, the more unfamiliar your particular traditions are likely to be to each other. So, the more fun you're going to have discovering them, explaining them, and trying to integrate them. We are all familiar with many rituals and traditions that coexist in America—from Shrove Tuesday to Superbowl Sunday. Some are ethnic or regional, some are religious or patriotic, but as Americans, we are free to enjoy them all, or not, as we please.

The most obvious traditions, of course, are related to ethnic backgrounds and religious observances, but other personal traditions have a special meaning or significance for those who honor them. You can even create your own customs, thus giving meaning to the unique history the two of you share. Here are some ideas:

- Celebrate odd anniversary dates (like you did in high school, remember?): the day you met, the first time you kissed, your "monthly" wedding anniversary.
- Make charity work part of a holiday celebration: serve turkey at a local soup kitchen on Thanksgiving, or get involved in a spring cleanup around Eastertime.
- Make "ritualistic" returns to scenes of special moments for the two of you: favorite restaurants, inns, vacation spots, parks, beaches, etc.
- Honor the changing seasons with some seasonal traditions of your own: try your hand at canning fruits and vegetables one weekend in the fall, take a winter ski trip to a favorite mountain lodge every January, or drive out to the country and pick wildflowers—baskets of them!—in late spring.
- Keep a guest book in your home so you have a record of friends and events over the years.
- Take photographs as a way of preserving memories; then, periodically, sit down and enjoy them together.
- Let *no* holiday go unremarked, and the more obscure the holiday, the better; decorate your home, even if only with thematic paper napkins at dinner, and exchange greeting cards, even if homemade. An occasion is only special if you make it so. (See more about "Celebrating Holidays" in Chapter 4.)

Handling Crises

Nobody can be truly prepared for a crisis when it comes, but it does seem especially unfortunate when newlyweds face traumas that would challenge the love and commitment of even long-married couples. "You hear terrible news all the time, but you never really think terrible things are going to happen to you," says Bonnie, looking back on her own ordeal. "But then they do, and you can't help but wonder why. It seems so unfair."

For Bonnie and Ray, the crisis began just eight months into their marriage when doctors discovered that Ray, only 25 years old, had testicular cancer. He had surgery immediately, but subsequent tests proved that the cancer was more pervasive than originally thought, so he had to have a more radical procedure. Ray was told to deposit his semen in a sperm bank before the second operation if he wished ever to have any natural children of his own.

"I was a basket case," Bonnie admits. "You just can't imagine what it's like to have your young, good-looking husband walk in the door one day and announce that he has cancer. You hear that word and you think, 'That's it. It's all over. I'm going to lose him.' And you are angry and sad and scared, all at the same time."

But she didn't lose him. Regular checkups have proven Ray to be cancer free for four years now, and—the best of all news—the couple has a new, healthy baby boy, their own son from insemination.

"After you've been through something like this, you learn to take nothing for granted in this life," Bonnie remarks. "And you certainly learn to put things in perspective, like you don't argue about stupid, ridiculous little things, or get hung up on the minor hassles of everyday life. In a way, I suppose you could say that Ray and I live a fuller life now, because we value every moment and every experience we have together."

Everything you go through together, both the good and the bad, builds a reservoir of shared history and emotional and spiritual strength. Bad experiences, though, may build that strength sooner simply because the two of you

---

What Other Couples Say . . .

"My father used to say that scar tissue is stronger than regular tissue," says one newlywed, "so once you survive a serious crisis, you're better equipped to handle anything else that comes your way."

Problem pregnancies, serious illness, family deaths, debilitating accidents, personal bankruptcy—we've heard it all from newlywed couples, and yes, catastrophe puts an unbelievable strain on the marriage. But, to a one, those who have come through disaster say that they bonded together as a couple sooner, and more deeply, than they might have otherwise, and that they have gained new insights into themselves and each other, and what really matters in life.

must unite against a common foe, the hardship. The trust you come to have and the mutual responsibility you assume for each other's well-being are the very essence of the marital bond.

"All those days and nights in the hospital, and then weeks of recuperation at home," Bonnie recalls, "and then a difficult pregnancy for me and more days and nights and weeks of mutual concern and support—all that time together really taught us who we were and what we were made of as a couple. And now that we know that, I don't think there's anything, not anything, that could threaten our love and devotion to each other. We're together—forever!"

Bonding Together

"Everybody is so concerned about finding the right person," one newlywed says. "What about finding the right attitude?"

Exactly. Building a marriage is about finding an attitude that works for your relationship, not against it. Workable attitudes will emphasize cooperation over competition, deference over domination, sharing over selfishness, interdependence over dependence. The right attitudes will create the right atmosphere, and the right atmosphere will turn your home into a haven from the pressures and conflicts of the outside world. The right attitude will ultimately turn you into the right person for each other.

Rev. Mark Connolly, a Catholic priest who counsels couples and who has produced a video guide to marriage (see Appendix), emphasizes the responsibility each spouse has for becoming the best he or she can be: "Success in marriage is not so much about finding the right partner as it is about *being* the right partner," he says.

Like any other vocation, marriage requires a dedication of purpose, a desire to become "good at the job." You do this by developing the skills and attributes that will allow each of you to find fulfillment and success in the partnership. All the things we've been talking about—realistic expectations, reasonable self-knowledge, a sense of humor, communication, intimacy, spirituality—are the tools that enable you to become good for yourself and for each other. And only then, when you are each pleased with who you are and confident and secure in your marital roles, can you transcend the individual self and become part of the other. Only then can you bond together as an inseparable whole.

Much has been written about the bonding that must take place between parent and child in order for that child to grow up healthy and secure. Isn't it logical, then, to assume that the same kind of bonding must occur first and foremost between the two partners in marriage? Otherwise, how could any two adults, coming together as most of us do as strangers, reasonably expect to stay together for a lifetime?

"Nothing is so special, so sacred as two people coming together to build a shared life," says Father Connolly. "Marriage is a process of growing together. Romance makes it happen, love makes it possible, and work makes it a reality."

So, when do you become those special people who are finally able, who have found the courage, to make the leap of faith in yourself and in each other? For some couples, particularly those who face unusual challenges early on as we've seen, that kind of unwavering trust in the permanence of their commitment happens in the first few years of marriage; for others, it may take a much longer time. But it will happen. And one day, perhaps at the oddest time, you will realize that it has happened to you.

> And stand together yet not too near together:
> For the pillars of the temple stand apart,
> And the oak tree and the cypress grow not in
> each other's shadow.
>
> —Gibran's *The Prophet*

Committing Forever

No one should marry, of course, without the commitment to try to make the marriage work. Even remarriage is a testament to the belief in the possibility of a lasting union. But there's no question that higher expectations of the marital relationship, more autonomy and choices for women, and the elimination of the stigma of divorce in society have all contributed to a more casual acceptance of the dissolution of a marriage.

The rocky periods of adjustment that most newlyweds experience can understandably undermine a couple's confidence in their ability to survive, but what's even worse is that by fretting over minor disagreements, couples miss the larger opportunity for growth. As Dr. Charles Cole of Iowa State University points out, the early married period of six to eighteen months is a couple's "most teachable moment." Dr. Cole, who has made the study of newlyweds the focus of his career, feels that six months or so into the marriage is the perfect time for couples to begin the work of developing the skills that will sustain them for a lifetime.

"Couples come to marriage with a high degree of satisfaction," he says. "They're in love. They've usually had no serious conflicts, so they don't even know what they need to know as a couple. But, once a few months have passed and some difficulties have erupted, then they are in an optimal learning curve; they are able to understand the need for problem-solving skills and to benefit most from counseling and advice."

Dr. Cole, and all the other marriage and family experts interviewed for this book, agree that more newlyweds should take advantage of couple workshops, support groups, and even private counseling early in their marriages before minor, routine problems become major, divisive issues. "Premarital programs get couples thinking about what their relationship means," Dr. Cole says, "but only intervention after the marriage can help a couple understand what their relationship really is and how it works. A willingness to seek that intervention, especially during periods of conflict, indicates a solid commitment to the marriage."

It comes as no surprise that couples who accept divorce as an option are more likely to exercise that option and to work less diligently at their marriages than those who express a firm resolve to make their unions last. Unfortunately, Western culture romanticizes love and marriage and attributes happiness and longevity more to "the luck" of having found the right person than to the work of having become the right partner. Don't let that myth undermine your ability to persevere in your relationship and your power to create the kind of lasting, loving union you deserve.

The Basic Needs of Happy Couples

Happy couples have needs, too. Here are the most basic ones to help assure that you and your relationship will thrive and grow.

Happy couples need

- To be accepted, faults and all, by each other and to be cherished, respected, and supported by their spouse in spite of imperfections
- Individual accomplishments that enhance self-worth and keep the balance of power in the relationship
- Uninterrupted time alone together, regularly, wherein each can focus on the other solely and completely
- Couple friends like themselves who have good marriages and with whom they can enjoy positive experiences
- Individual friends with whom to enjoy personal interests and activities independent of their spouse
- A shared history of positive experiences and meaningful traditions on which to build a vision and a purpose for the future
- A sense of humor
- An ability to adapt, change, and grow with changing circumstances
- A belief in the permanence of their union

Determining a Lifestyle

When we talk about lifestyle, we usually mean the kinds of cars people drive, the homes they live in, or the friends they have. Such things, taken together, become symbolic of the way one lives, or would like to live. We begin to identify and classify people accordingly as "jet-setters," "fast-trackers," or "just plain folks."

As we mature, each of us gradually assumes the attitudes and accoutrements of a lifestyle that we feel best reflects and projects our image of ourselves. Sometimes that image has been formed by the family we grew up in; sometimes not. Sometimes the image is born out of educational and professional associations; sometimes not. Sometimes the image is consistent with the reality of our circumstances; sometimes not.

Regardless of how our lifestyle develops, the way we choose to live, or the style of life to which we aspire, serves as a very real indication of what's most important to us—our basic values. Since the two of you have made the decision to live this life together, it's important that you have shared values.

Values and Priorities

Our values, and the choices we make because of them, emanate from a basic philosophy of life. Taken together, philosophy, values, and choices translate into a visible "lifestyle." If we look at life as a never-ending party, then we are more likely to indulge in material pleasures, leisure activities, and the things money can buy. On the other hand, if we're more pessimistic and see life as a never-ending struggle, then we tend to value the tools of survival: hard work, status and power, financial security. Few of us live entirely at one extreme or the other of our beliefs, and our view of life can be changed dramatically by broadened experience and new influences on our thinking. More education, more travel, a larger circle of friends, different regional customs—all can expose us to other values and ways of doing things.

Even without that exposure, priorities can change as circumstances change, as a goal is met or a need is fulfilled. Someone who has faced great hardship in childhood, for example, might devote young adulthood to the almost compulsive accumulation of wealth, only to turn around and give it all away in later years. As situations change, so might priorities. Thus, making lifestyle choices

---

❧❧   DO YOU SEE YOURSELF HERE?   ❧❧

- Do you come from markedly different socioeconomic backgrounds?
- Does one of you have significantly higher material and social expectations than the other?
- Do your tastes and expectations far exceed your financial and social realities?
- Do the two of you argue over the quality vs. quantity (of style) issue?
- Is one of you often made to feel inferior or socially inept by the other's family or friends?
- Are you unsure of your entertaining skills, or generally uncomfortable in social situations?
- Is one of you jealous of the time the other spends with his or her friends or family members?

For discussions of all your "yes" answers, read on.

---

requires that we periodically reorder and rethink our values and make new distinctions between what we simply want and what we really need.

"Ruel and I joke about our champagne tastes," laughs Barbara as she sorts through a pile of cruise folders in anticipation of the couple's upcoming vacation. "I really don't know where we get it from. We were both raised by single parents, so it's not as though we grew up in affluence. But, I guess you don't have to be rich to appreciate the finer things."

Ruel and Barbara both have lucrative jobs, and together they earn a substantial income. They work hard and, consequently, they feel they have a right to the fruits of that labor. They enjoy good food, luxurious places, and pretty things. In short, Ruel and Barbara both like "the good life," maybe precisely because they didn't have much of it growing up. At this particular time, they can afford to pursue it. They don't have heavy family obligations, outstanding education loans, or children yet, so a little self-indulgence is not out of line.

Even so, the couple is sensible enough to realize that they could easily find themselves living way beyond their means if they didn't make choices and control their impulses. For example, they don't kid themselves about their ability to economize when they travel, so they choose to take a vacation every other year instead of every year.

"We decided we would rather have one big trip than two smaller ones," Ruel explains. "Actually, we find we're sort of like that in everything. I'd rather have one good suit than two or three cheaper ones."

Barbara nods in agreement. "Yeah, one good piece of jewelry rather than a whole lot of costume."

Ruel and Barbara's attitudes reflect not only a similar approach to making lifestyle choices, but also similar underlying goals and values. Both believe in financial responsibility, but both also go for quality over quantity. Knowing that as a couple they have to work to keep what seems like conflicting values in check, Ruel and Barbara are able to help each other make reasonable lifestyle choices as they go along.

Setting Mutual Goals

Knowing what you value most in life gives you a direction for the future and the ability to set goals for both the short and the long term. Those goals will ultimately determine what kind of couple you're going to become and how you're going to be perceived by others. Will you be very social, warm, and friendly, a couple whose doors are always open to everyone? Or, will you be perhaps a bit more formal and reserved, a couple who values intellectual pursuits and personal integrity over multitudes of friends and a full social calendar?

The lifestyle choices you make now will influence your future together. The closer you are in values, obviously, the less conflict you will have over these choices and the easier your existence as a couple will be. Furthermore, you will be able to support each other in ways you otherwise might not be willing to if you didn't believe in the same things. If both of you place a high value on education, for instance, then one of you will be more willing to sacrifice and support the other if he or she decides to pursue a graduate degree.

Following is a list of commonly held values. Which ones are important to you? Do you and your spouse share the most important ones?

> social status/class
> personal integrity/reputation
> health/fitness
> physical appearance
> material comforts
> aesthetics
> cultural pursuits (theater, art, literature, etc.)
> financial security
> wealth/power
> family ties and traditions
> spiritual/religious beliefs
> friends/social network
> education/learning
> social activism (charity work, ecology, peace, etc.)
> patriotism/political ideology
> satisfying work/career success

Note that these values, in and of themselves, are neither positive nor negative. Rather, it is how they are pursued, and to what extent and for what reason, that invites moral judgment.

In order for the two of you to work toward the same things, you have to be honest about what you value and what you want out of life. If having nice things and surrounding yourself with beauty, art, and culture is important to you, then be sure your spouse understands and appreciates that before you invest big bucks in a painting for the living room.

Sharing the same goals does not mean, however, that you have to share exactly the same taste or that each of you has to follow the same pursuits. Marriage is a partnership, remember? Decisions may be mutual, but each of you is enabled to reach some personal goals and accomplishments precisely because you have the added support of the other.

Ideally, personal achievements and satisfactions make life better and happier for you both, but only when the two of you have agreed on their pursuit for the common good.

The Taste Test

Sharing the same values and lifestyle goals cannot always guarantee that two people will make the same choices, especially in matters of taste. Music, art, literature, dress, food, home furnishings, architecture—even connoisseurs and scholars argue about which is the very best from among selections that are, in terms of worth and quality, essentially the same. Ultimately, it boils down to a purely subjective response; for the most part, matters of taste are matters of opinion.

Back to Barbara and Ruel. "There was this couch I just loved for our living room," she recalls. "I'll admit that it was expensive, but even Ruel had to agree that it was very well constructed and that it would last for years."

That, as it turns out, was the crux of the problem. "I couldn't believe that Barbara liked this thing," he says. "It had these big, gloppy flowers all over it—

What Other Couples Say . . .

Money may not buy happiness, but there's no question that having enough of it contributes to marital well-being. Why? Because money allows couples freedom of choice, in purchasing goods and services, for instance, and takes the stress out of some major decisions, like having a family or buying a house. Statistics indicate that divorce rates are lower among higher-income couples.

Authors/researchers Dr. Sue Simring, a psychotherapist, and Dr. Steven Simring, a psychiatrist, have also found that education is positively related to marital stability and happiness. People with college degrees have significantly lower divorce rates than those with barely a high school education, presumably because they are more sophisticated about relationships and more adept at interpersonal skills. More education may also translate into higher-paying, higher-status careers, which also positively affect marital stability.

I hate flowers anyway—and the couch weighed a ton. I just knew I'd have to look at it and lug it around for the rest of my life."

Ultimately, the two compromised. They bought a smaller, plainer, well-made couch that will relocate easily to other rooms and other homes, and Barbara satisfied her desire for a floral pattern with draperies. "I'm still not too crazy about the print on the drapes," Ruel says, "but it's okay because the rest of the room offsets it."

"Who notices the rest of the room when the draperies are so spectacular!" teases Barbara.

You can't really argue about matters of taste, although unfortunately lots of couples do. It's a pointless argument because there's seldom any real logic behind why one likes or dislikes something. Often when the person expressing the preference is asked why he feels as he does, he'll simply say, "Because I just do." That's because many of our preferences have been inculcated by our backgrounds or conditioned out of sheer habit. They are so ingrained that we don't even think about them until someone asks us to. We think we prefer toast with scrambled eggs and coffee in the morning, for example, because that's what we've always had, but we might like English muffins as well, or better, if we only gave them a try.

As a couple, you'll want to push the limits of your own individual experience and let your combined talents and tastes complement each other as you decorate your home and make lifestyle choices. In some instances, one of you might defer a selection to the other because he or she, for whatever reason, is in a better position to make a more knowledgeable choice. Perhaps one of you has a more sensitive eye for design or for the nuances of color, while the other has more knowledge and appreciation for structural soundness or mechanical precision.

Building a mutual lifestyle requires a willingness to try new things, to be receptive to new ideas, and to respect the contributions of your partner. No two people will ever have exactly the same tastes and habits in everything, but you can always find ways to integrate preferences into a style of life comfortable for both of you. (See more about style and taste in Chapter 6.)

Lifestyles of the Not-So-Rich and Famous

Okay, time to be honest. Each of you should take the quiz separately and choose the *one* answer that best completes your initial response to the statement. Then compare your answers. Which of your lifestyle goals and values are in synch? Minor differences are to be expected, but if you discover major areas of disagreement, you'd better settle them fast, before you have to decide how to spend that first million!

1. My idea of a great evening is
   a.   dinner for two at an elegant restaurant
   b.   pizza and beer at home in front of the TV
   c.   an informal get-together with friends or family
   d.   a lavish party with new and interesting people
2. What I most like to do in my spare time is
   a.   read
   b.   watch TV
   c.   pursue a hobby or favorite activity
   d.   see friends/family
3. What I most dislike doing in my spare time is
   a.   housework/yardwork
   b.   sitting in front of the TV
   c.   shopping
   d.   seeing people
4. If I can't go first class when I travel, I would
   a.   rather not go at all
   b.   go economy class but complain all the way
   c.   happily go economy class because I've never traveled any other way
   d.   certainly go economy class because I think first-class frills are a waste of money
5. I judge a restaurant by
   a.   the prices on the menu
   b.   the quality of the food and service
   c.   the atmosphere and ambience
   d.   what others say about it
6. If I won a $10 million lottery, the first thing I would do would be to
   a.   quit my job
   b.   buy a new house or car
   c.   give an extravagant gift to someone I love
   d.   invest the money for the future
7. When I meet someone new, I am most easily turned off by
   a.   an unattractive physical appearance
   b.   inappropriate dress
   c.   incorrect language usage
   d.   name-dropping and pretentiousness
8. When I go to someone's home, I am most conscious of
   a.   the neighborhood and size of the house
   b.   the decor and style of furnishings
   c.   the state of housekeeping and clutter
   d.   the atmosphere of hospitality
9. Were I to throw a big party, my guests would be
   a.   friends and neighbors
   b.   business and professional associates
   c.   mostly family members
   d.   a hodgepodge of friends, family, and associates

10. The possession that means the most to me is
    a. something of sentimental value, but not of much monetary value
    b. something of sentimental value that is also valuable, such as a family heirloom
    c. something I worked for, such as a car or a fur coat
    d. nothing; I'm not into possessions
11. To me, being successful means
    a. being at the top of my business or profession
    b. having enough money to live the way I choose and not having to worry about it
    c. being happy and being loved
    d. having it all!
12. If the devil were to tempt me with one great gift, I would be most easily seduced by
    a. wealth
    b. power
    c. fame
    d. beauty

Pursuing Interests and Hobbies

The best advice about interests and hobbies is that you both need some—some you can pursue together, and some you pursue alone or with friends. Leisure activities allow us to relax and have fun, and often provide an outlet for enjoying the aptitudes and talents that we don't use in our professional lives. That's important because none of us is one dimensional.

Chances are that some shared interests—sports, cooking, collecting, etc.— are what brought the two of you together in the first place. You should continue to enjoy those pastimes together, maybe even consider expanding your skills for fuller participation in what could become a lifelong source of mutual satisfaction and enjoyment. Who knows? You might discover hidden talents, or even opportunities for a new business venture.

If you didn't have outside interests or other passions before marriage, now is the time to develop some—an abiding passion for your spouse is not enough. Remember Janice and Jerry, the couple who suffered from the "Honeymoon Hangover"? Part of their problem was Janice's lack of independent interests and her need to be part of everything Jerry did.

"With so little time together, I found myself jealous of his softball games, which I really didn't enjoy that much, or resentful of the time he spent in the gym with his friends," she admits. "Then I realized that I was really jealous of the fact that Jerry had outside interests, which I didn't have, and that if I was busy enjoying myself without him sometimes, I wouldn't be so angry at him for having a good time without me."

These days, Janice is becoming "a gallivanting gourmet," as Jerry puts it. She has taken several cooking classes and has made new friends who are interested in food and wine. Her new acquaintances and new experiences have, in turn, given her more social confidence, so that she and Jerry now entertain more at home and go out more with a wider variety of people.

Unfortunately, leisure activities are often the first things to be eliminated when time and money are tight. Don't let that happen. If your financial resources are slim, develop hobbies like camping, sewing, or refinishing furniture, activities that are not only relatively inexpensive, but that might actually save you money. If time is a problem, look for pursuits that can be enjoyed anytime you have a few minutes or while you're doing something else, things like listening to books on tape while you're driving or taking an exercise class during your lunch break.

Hobbies and leisure activities are not frivolous pursuits; they are vehicles for necessary relaxation, meaningful companionship, and better mental health.

Couple and Community

"My father-in-law has been active in the community all his life," Jody explains. "United Way, Knights of Columbus, Rotary Club, Small Business Association—you name it. So when my husband's mother said to me one night, before we were married, that I should take note of how Augie's dad was with all his clubs and organizations and take care not to let Augie and myself fall into the same patterns, I wasn't really sure what she meant. After all, being a 'pillar of the community' is usually thought of as desirable."

Within six months after they were married, Jody understood. Already, Augie was coaching a boys' basketball team, spearheading a major project for the Jaycees, serving on an advisory board for the local men's shelter, and involved in several different activities at church. He was out almost every night doing something.

"Not that what he was doing wasn't worthwhile," Jody is quick to add, "but we weren't doing any of it together. All I kept thinking was that if we were leading parallel lives already as newlyweds, how would it be when we had children and there were more and more activities and obligations to attend to?"

When the couple sat down to talk about this, Augie had to admit that his house had been like a railway station when he was growing up. His father had set an expectation of involvement, and so everybody ran in different directions: dad to civic affairs, kids to sports and school activities, and mom to church and PTA. They left notes on the refrigerator door and rarely sat down to dinner together.

In contrast, Jody realized that while her parents, too, had encouraged school, church, and community participation, lots of activities involved the entire family, and her mom and dad joined many things as a couple. Moreover, dinnertime had been sacred in her household.

Studies have shown that being embedded in a social network is "critical to both marital satisfaction and marital stability" (Kurdek, 1047). Couples need not only each other and their immediate families, but also a wide network of friends, colleagues, and coworkers with whom to interact and to derive mutual support and self-esteem. This network is largely created through business and professional associations, civic and community activities, religious and charitable organizations, clubs for athletics or special interests, and active involvement in the affairs of the neighborhood, the workplace, and the schools. When family members and/or old friends are not nearby or accessible, it is even more important to cultivate a social support system from this kind of community network.

BUT, and this is a big but, you have to safeguard time to spend alone with each other and time for the enjoyment of mutual pursuits. Otherwise, Jody's fear is well founded: what will happen when your life gets even more complicated than it is now? Being a newlywed in a community is like being a freshman in college: everyone wants you to join, but it's easy to get overextended. No doubt both of you work full-time and have some time demands from your careers. You may already be active in professional groups or other organizations from your single days. If you have family nearby, you will need to plan time with them. The question becomes, then, how much time and energy is left, and where will it be best spent?

Certainly, you'll want to establish yourselves as a couple in the community, and there is no question that civic or charitable work creates tremendous personal rewards and satisfactions. But go slowly at first and look for activities the two of you can do together. Decide on one or two avenues of participation you would both enjoy, perhaps through your church or synagogue, or a political party, and don't let yourselves get overscheduled. You can always increase your involvement as time goes by, but it is extremely difficult to extricate yourself once committed.

By the way, Augie did extricate himself from several of his commitments, and the couple has decided to concentrate on mostly church activities for now, at least some of which overlap. They have also agreed to one night out a week, separately, for their own pursuits, whether that's dinner with personal friends or attendance at a meeting. "At least we're monitoring our time and thinking about our commitments these days," Jody says. "You don't have to become a 'pillar of the community' overnight."

Old Friends and New

At different times, your husband will play different roles in your life: husband, father, lover, son, partner, and friend. And, you will do the same for him. But isn't it a lot to ask one person to stand ready to wear any or all of those hats at any given moment? Of course it is. That's why we have friends.

Marriage is a new stage of life. You will meet new people, try new things, acquire new responsibilities. Yet, even though you'll now have your very best friend in permanent residence, being married doesn't eliminate the value of other relationships. When it comes to marital friendships, then, the well-known advice still applies: "Make new friends, but keep the old. One is silver, the other is gold."

There is room, and need, for both in your married lifestyle. Old friends validate us; like family, they are there over time and distance to support and sustain us regardless of the changes that occur from day to day. We may not be able to see them as often as we would like, and we may have to make an extra effort to keep the bonds intact, but old friends are part of who we are, part of the personal identity we bring to marriage. Old friends are extremely important.

New friends, on the other hand, enliven us; they reflect what's current in our lives, our changing interests, activities, and circumstances. Most newlyweds develop new friends, usually other couples like themselves, who are also adjusting to a new way of life. Making friends as a couple, then, is also important because it reinforces the shared history that the two of you are beginning to build together. Like schoolmates, some of the friends you make as early marrieds will be with you over a lifetime.

Time for Everyone

The great difficulty in developing and maintaining friendships in marriage is time. The simple truth is that you'll have less of it. In addition to all your old responsibilities of job and home and self, you will have additional obligations to your new spouse and family that will also compete for attention. Those pressures, in turn, heighten the natural inclination for couples in love to be selfish, to want to spend the precious little spare time they have alone with each other.

The two of you will need to examine the role of others in your life and to discuss your personal feelings with honesty, trust, and understanding. You will also have to recognize that no one person in a relationship, even a husband or a wife, can possibly fill another's every emotional, social, professional, and intellectual need. To expect that kind of exclusivity and intensity from a spouse is to expect too much of the marital partnership.

Thus, a healthy circle of friends contributes to the strength of the marriage. As with every other mutual lifestyle choice, however, the two of you will have to work together to find the right social mix of old and new, personal and professional friends. You may have to compromise. He may have to spend an occasional evening with a business colleague of yours who bores him, or you may have to act as a gracious hostess for his crazy college roommate for a weekend

---

What Other Couples Say . . .

Among the sources of emotional support that newlyweds name and count on, personal friends are mentioned as second in importance only to the spouse. In third place is one's immediate family of origin (mother, father, sister, brother), then the relatives (aunts, uncles, cousins, grandparents, etc.), then in-laws (the spouse's family), and finally coworkers (Kurdek, 1050).

visit. But these are small concessions to make for each other's happiness and well-being.

Years from now, as you speak of the mutual friends who have become so special to you both, you'll be glad that you always took the time to share your life together with other people. And your relationship will be the richer because of it.

Your Social Image

"Martin's family is *very* social, I mean like yacht club, garden party type social," says Amanda, "and so are a lot of Martin's old friends. He went to a New England prep school, was into sailing and tennis and soccer, all the stuff families like his encourage their children to do. It's not that his family and friends are snobs or anything, because they're not, really. It's just that his experience growing up was so different from mine. Sometimes I still feel out-classed around all of them."

Amanda's feelings are not unreasonable because she and Martin are from markedly different socioeconomic backgrounds: he's from an upper-middle-class New England family that, while not enormously wealthy, is affluent enough, and well enough connected, to have afforded their children a somewhat privileged upbringing. She, on the other hand, comes from an urban, working-class background, and was the first in her family to obtain a college degree. The couple met at an Ivy League university, in fact, where Martin was paying full tuition and Amanda was on full scholarship.

Similar values and interests, even mutual friends, brought the two together in college, so they are obviously not that different "on the inside, where it counts," as Amanda puts it. But, external tastes and expectations, "the social trappings," are another story, as the couple found out when they began planning their wedding.

"We decided to plan and pay for the wedding ourselves, as a way of striking a balance between the obvious social differences of the two families, but there ended up being clashes anyway," Amanda recalls. "Martin's family expected certain things that we just couldn't afford to do, and my family accused me of 'putting on airs' with some of our choices. Eventually, we compromised by having the ceremony at my old neighborhood church in the city followed by a garden reception later in the day at my in-laws' home in the suburbs. But that proved to be both inconvenient and unwise. We should have stuck to our original plans and kept the wedding on neutral territory all around."

It is interesting, but maybe not surprising, that Martin and Amanda's wedding experience taught them their first important social lesson for married life: establish your own style and stick to it. This is especially true if you come from different socioeconomic backgrounds, or if you have a broad spectrum of friends. Unless you plan to spend your lives as social chameleons, there will just never be a way to please all the people all the time, so your only recourse is to please yourselves. Decide how you want to live and what your priorities are, and then set about building that lifestyle.

You've probably begun to do that already through your bridal gift registry and home furnishings selections. If you registered fine china, crystal, and sterling silver, for instance, then you obviously value a certain graciousness of style, even a degree of formality, and you expect to live and entertain in a way that uses these fine accessories, at least on occasion. Then again, maybe the last things on earth you could ever imagine needing or wanting would be a silver platter or a demitasse coffee set, so you chose to acquire more affordable, practical items, such as cookware, appliances, and everyday dinnerware.

Between your own registry choices and the wedding gifts you received, a very clear statement has been made about the style of life you expect, and are expected, to lead. It would be wise for the two of you to talk about those implications, particularly as they affect your relationships with family, friends, and professional associates.

Five Frequent Faux Pas

Etiquette is just plain common sense, as noted in the rules that follow. Break one of these and it's a real social blunder. Best advice: DON'T!

1. **Respond to an invitation:** R.S.V.P. on an invitation means you *must* respond, promptly, either by phone, handwritten note, or by mailing an enclosed response card if one has been included. If you are issued an oral invitation and have to check your dates first, be sure to get back promptly with a reply. It is always a serious faux pas to fail to respond to an invitation.

2. **Be on time:** There are certain functions for which you simply *cannot* be late. They are: weddings, funerals, a sit-down dinner, and the theater, opera, or other artistic performance. To come in late is not only rude, but inconsiderate.

3. **Write thank-you notes:** Handwritten thank-you notes, not printed cards, *must* be sent for every gift, including those from relatives, close friends, and business associates. This means for birthdays, Christmas/Hanukkah, anniversaries, and all other major occasions when gifts are given or sent. It is also good manners to write or call in appreciation for a previous dinner engagement or other hospitality. Saying "thank you" is perhaps the most neglected rule of etiquette, and yet, in a simple way, it is the most important rule of all.

4. **Know gift protocol:** Gifts are usually expected for birthday parties, showers, weddings, anniversaries, retirements, and house warmings, but you do not have to send a gift to an event which you do not attend, although you certainly may if you wish. It is never proper to tell someone what to give you as a gift, or even to suggest that they give a gift at all, because gifts are exactly that: freely offered tokens of affection that are not to be demanded or expected.

5. **Dress appropriately:** Being underdressed is *always* preferable to being overdressed, so don't break out the sequins unless you're sure others will be wearing the same. "Black tie" or "Black tie invited" means a tuxedo for the men and formal or semiformal attire for the women; men may also wear a dark business suit and a white shirt to a black tie affair, but never a sports coat or blazer.

Bridging Gaps

It is not a matter of any one style or image being better than another so much as it is what is appropriate to who you are and the social setting in which you find yourselves. And that social setting, and the attendant social obligations, can also change. What is acceptable, and expected, from you as newlyweds living in a one-bedroom apartment with no furniture will not do ten years from now. A job promotion, a larger home, a broader circle of personal and professional friends, a family of your own—all will affect your social status and the image you project, and have to live up to.

No matter how casual and laid-back your everyday lifestyle is right now, you can't afford to be a social clod. There will be times, such as formal parties or business affairs, that necessitate a certain style and decorum. Just as with most other tastes, habits, and behaviors, the social graces are largely learned at home. If you were raised setting tables for dinner parties and preparing to entertain houseguests, then you'll be comfortable meeting, greeting, and dining when the occasions arise. If not, you'll have to get a good etiquette book and study up when necessary.

That doesn't mean you're being a fake, either. Personal charm and distinctive style evolve from blending one's own background and traditions into present social circumstances. If you have "married up" so to speak, as Amanda feels she has, or moved up the social ladder because of educational or career success, then you'll have to work on your social skills until you are comfortable in the milieu in which you find yourself. Proper etiquette, after all, means helping others feel comfortable and welcome, and you can't do that until you, yourself, are. And that has to be genuine.

Entertaining Style

Nothing will establish your image as a couple, or cement your relationships with others, more than the manner and the frequency with which you entertain. If your home is open and your hearts are warm, you are assured a loyal and loving group of friends, relatives, and even colleagues with whom to share the landmarks, and the lows, in life.

There are all sorts of ways to entertain, from impromptu potluck suppers with the neighbors, to elegant, sit-down dinners for the boss. You might treat friends or clients to an evening out, at the theater perhaps, or a sporting event, or you might simply invite them to meet you at the movies and then come to your house for dessert and coffee afterward. Entertaining doesn't have to be expensive, nor do you have to pay for everything just because you initiate the ideas.

These days, most couples choose to entertain at home, not only because they can more easily keep expenses in line, but also because planning parties and get-togethers at home is a very creative and satisfying activity. Those who have the space and the know-how often prefer to entertain even business clients at home. Socially experienced couples know that offering the hospitality and intimacy of one's own home is the highest compliment, and they take a great deal of pride and pleasure in their ability to be gracious hosts.

Besides all that, entertaining at home is just plain fun, and it gives you a chance to use some of those great wedding gifts! The more you entertain, the better you'll get at it and the more social savvy you'll develop. Pretty soon, the two of you will be as fine a team as any caterers, and the flow of planning, cooking, serving, and cleanup tasks will become automatic. And so will the compliments of your guests.

So, go ahead. Be adventurous and let the spirit of generosity move you toward discovering your own unique style. Use the following "Easy Entertaining Guide" to inspire you and get you started.

Easy Entertaining Guide

The Who

Every great hostess knows that the real secret to the success of any party, large or small, is the guest list. The right mix of people will generate its own excitement so that guests actually entertain themselves; the wrong mix can be woefully dull—even deadly.

Basically, your guest list is going to depend on who you like, who you owe, and what the occasion is. Then, there are the practical considerations: how many people can your home accommodate, how much do you want to spend, and how much time and work are you willing to invest? Once all that is determined, consider the following:

A Large Affair
35 to 40 guests, and up
Written or printed invitations, depending on formality
Options: brunch, lunch or dinner buffet, barbecue, tea/dessert, cocktail party, open house
Advantages: varied guest list—may mix family, friends, professionals, of various ages, occupations, interests; festive mood makes party seem to run itself; can reciprocate many invitations with just one event and can combine "business with pleasure"
Disadvantages: demands sufficient space and service equipment; requires considerable advanced planning; can be costly, depending on menu; should have some service help, such as bartender or waiters; offers little opportunity for in-depth conversation

A Medium Affair
15 to 25 guests
Written or telephoned invitations

Options: brunch, lunch or dinner buffet, picnic or patio barbecue, potluck, cocktail party, desserts and coffee

Advantages: easier to plan and can usually do without service help; may invite a mixed group because guests will cluster by interests; more intimate conversation possible

Disadvantages: still have to consider space, traffic patterns, and service equipment; guest list can't be quite as broad as for a larger affair; can be costly, depending on menu

A Small Affair

4 to 10 guests

Telephoned or written invitations, depending on formality

Options: sit-down or buffet brunch, lunch or dinner, patio cookout, potluck, dessert and coffee; ideal size for elegant dinner party.

Advantages: lends itself to impromptu planning and informal style; can do alone without help or great expense; intimate group, great conversation; can plan a more exotic or involved menu

Disadvantages: must carefully select guest list for compatibility and complementary traits, such as talkers and listeners, similar interests or connections; can be a lot of work, and expense, if done as a formal sit-down dinner

Hosting Hints

- It's good manners to reciprocate an invitation within a few months of your having been entertained, but you don't have to reciprocate in kind. That is, if you were invited to a dinner party, you don't have to entertain with dinner in return. Instead, you might ask the couple to join you at an art exhibit or museum opening, then treat to coffee and cake afterward.

- Show respect for cultural or religious customs by knowing your guests and providing alternatives: meatless entrees for Catholics on Fridays in Lent, for instance, or nonalcoholic beverages for those who do not drink. If guests choose not to honor their own customs or restrictions, that's their business, but you shouldn't put them on the spot in your home.

- If you regularly entertain foreign visitors, study up. Even though, technically, American customs prevail when foreigners visit here, you wouldn't want to inadvertently offend a guest in your home. Furthermore, a small acknowledgment of a foreign visitor's custom or taste in the way of food, fare, or decoration, is most gracious, and will be appreciated.

- Anyone invited to your home should be specifically invited with his or her own phone call or written invitation. In other words, don't say, "Oh, by the way, bring your mother."

- Some people still smoke. Provisions should be made for that, and smokers should be made aware of what those provisions are. Most smokers are not rude and will gladly comply with your requests.

- Don't let anyone leave your home inebriated. Make sure there is a designated driver, or insist that the inebriated person spend the night on the couch!

What to Serve

Most home entertaining centers around food. So your choices for entertaining include breakfast, brunch, lunch, afternoon tea, cocktails, dinner, dessert and coffee, and midnight supper. How you choose to deliver this fare is, of course, up to you. (See next section.)

There are two schools of thought about cooking for a crowd: one school says that you should never make any dish for company that you haven't tried before; the other says that, if you are a somewhat experienced cook and your guests are good friends, there is nothing wrong with trying out something new for a party. It all depends on the confidence you have in yourself—and your cookbook.

Food Preparation

One big secret to successful entertaining is choosing dishes that can be prepared in advance, maybe even prepared well in advance and frozen, so that you are less harried at the event itself and can enjoy your guests. Casseroles (tuna, chicken, vegetarian), one-dish meals (chili, beef stew, lasagne), and roasted meats (turkey, ham, roast beef) are favorites because they virtually cook themselves while guests enjoy cocktails and hors d'oeuvres.

Another popular idea that makes entertaining easier and fun is to let your guests participate in food preparation, such as by making their own omelettes or assembling tacos or sundaes, or even cooking their own burgers on the grill. The food becomes the event and all you have to do is wash, chop, and trim all the ingredients and have them conveniently arranged. That, along with prepared salads and side dishes, can all be done in advance.

For a really informal evening, how about a "potluck supper"? The traditional version of this old-time favorite means asking guests to literally bring their leftovers at the end of the week; a more modern version is to plan and coordinate a simple menu, asking each guest to bring one of the items on it. Either way, potluck is just the kind of casual setting ideal for playing cards or watching old movies.

Then, too, you can always consider making some dishes and buying others already prepared. These days, with the proliferation of gourmet takeout and delivery services from some of the finest restaurants and specialty food markets, you can purchase almost anything your hearts, or palettes, desire. And, if you really want to pull out all the stops, you can even engage a caterer to come into your home and do all the work for you.

From dinner for two to a bash for fifty or more, the major considerations in choosing a menu are time, money, the tastes of your guests, and your own culinary expertise. Here are some cost-saving measures that can help you plan.

Food Economy

• Learn to shop for specials and buy in bulk; for instance, when chickens or steaks are featured, buy several and freeze them. That way, when guests drop in or you decide to have an impromptu party, you'll have your menu on hand.

- Fruit platters, cheese trays, or vegetable crudities are easy to do yourself, even if time consuming; buying such labor-intensive items is proportionately more expensive, so your entertaining dollars are better spent elsewhere.
- Spending a few extra pennies for "gourmet preparation" of a standard item, such as a rolled veal roast stuffed with spinach and cheese or a trimmed and decorated crown roast of pork, can make sense. The difficult part of the preparation, and the part that takes some know-how, is already done, so all you have to do to look like an accomplished chef is to cook it.
- Buy wines and beer by the case. It's cheaper that way, and you'll have it on hand.
- Plan menus with seasonal availability in mind. Fruits and vegetables will not only be cheaper, but they'll be of better quality.
- When you're in the mood to bake, bake two pies, or cakes, or loaves of bread, and freeze one. Essentially, you'll be doing the same amount of work, but you'll build a reserve of special items for entertaining later.
- If you cook or entertain frequently, consider purchasing a small additional refrigerator or freezer. For you, this could be a worthwhile investment.

How to Serve

The buffet is the greatest idea to come to the kitchen since home-baked bread! Any party can be done in buffet style, and many guests actually prefer serving themselves. The buffet can be elegant and formal, such as one sparkling with crystal and silver for a Christmas Eve supper, or informal and fun, such as cold cuts and salads laid out on the kitchen counter for Super Bowl Sunday. An inviting buffet can be situated almost anywhere—on a dining table, a sideboard, or even a countertop. Just be sure that the surface is large enough to contain everything you'll need for the number of guests, and that traffic can flow smoothly and easily.

Without a banquet-sized dining table and help to serve, most hosts/hostesses have to rely on the buffet when serving a meal for ten guests or more. Depending on your menu, much of the work can be done in advance, and cleanup is quick and easy, especially if you're using paper products.

For a large buffet (40 or more guests), arrange the table (Figure 1) so that guests can start at both ends, usually on opposite sides, and work their way toward the center. Ends of the table should mirror each other, with plates stacked and flatware arranged below the main courses. Diners move toward the middle of the table, where vegetables, salads, sauces, and condiments are placed. Napkins may be artfully arranged there so guests pick them up as they leave.

For a smaller buffet (Figure 2), the table is generally arranged on one side only from one end to the other. Beverages are more conveniently served from a different location, and soups, desserts, or other special courses may require their own separate stations. Just use common sense and be aware of traffic patterns when planning any buffet, large or small.

For formal, sit-down dining (Figure 3), begin by setting the service plates, if you're using them, or the dinner plates, if you're not. Distance between them

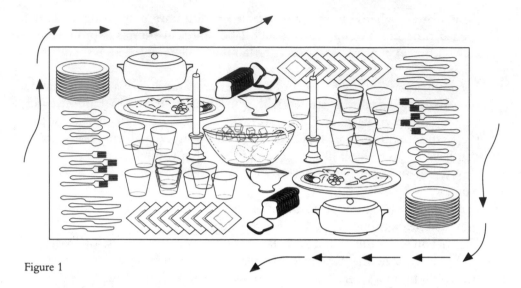

Figure 1

should be 24 inches from center to center. Flatware is arranged on either side with the first to be used farthest from the plate: the salad fork and dinner fork on the left; soup spoon, then knife placed with the cutting edge facing in on the right. Napkins, folded, are placed on the table to the left of the outside fork.

The bread and butter plate, used for luncheon or less formal dining, goes directly above the place fork on the left with the butter knife resting across it. The water goblet is situated squarely above the knife on the right, with champagne, and red and/or white wine glasses forming a triangle to the right. The salad plate usually sits to the left of the dinner plate, though according to strictest etiquette, the salad should be present on the service plate when diners seat themselves if it is to be a first course, or brought in separately after soup or fish if a subsequent course. The cup and saucer are set to the right of the dessert plate when that course is served.

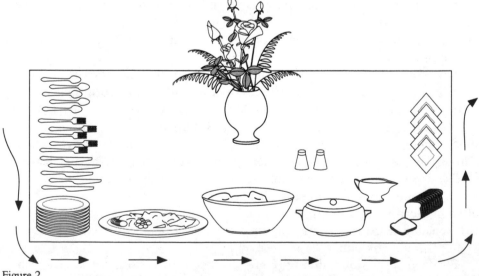

Figure 2

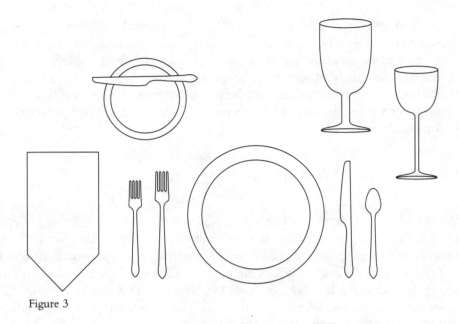

Figure 3

For especially important dinners and advice regarding multiple course service and the placement of other tabletop items, consult a reliable etiquette book.

Table Decorating Ideas
Edible centerpieces, like a bountiful cascade of fresh fruit or an aromatic arrangement of spices and herbs, are pleasing on any table. Flowers and candles are lovely adornments, too, but you need not limit your choices to them alone. Use your imagination and look around you when designing a tabletop to capture a mood. Figurines and collectibles, dried wood and dolls, cooking utensils and colored ribbon, almost anything can be fashioned into attractive and unusual table accents.

Think of your table linens, too, as a background for the drama of beautiful settings and brilliant conversations. Whether formal or informal, by candlelight or daylight, your linens should echo the mood, not shout it.

For Atmosphere and Ambience
- Use your beautiful china, crystal, and silver, even for informal affairs. The great advantage of owning quality items is that they are so versatile and adaptable.
- Take advantage of the many gorgeous paper products available today. They can be very elegant, and are always acceptable for large crowds. (Do not, however, mix paper products with fine crystal and silver.) Buy paper goods on sale or at warehouse outlets so you'll have them on hand.
- Renting can be costly. If you entertain frequently, consider purchasing inexpensive glassware and flatware just for parties. Perhaps you could even purchase sets in partnership with a close friend or relative; that way, you'll be able to borrow each other's for a larger service.

- Colored bedsheets, hemmed to size, make wonderful tablecloths and liners under lace covers. Because they are so large, and seamless, sheets are one of the best fabric buys around. You can also make matching napkins.
- Make an inventory of your most useful service plates, pitchers, and platters, and keep the list handy. This will help you remember what you have when planning a party, and allow you to pick up additional service pieces when you see them on sale.

When and Why to Entertain

Anytime is a good time for a party. Of course, there are all the obvious occasions: holidays, anniversaries, birthdays, graduations, and other special events. But then there are just ordinary days and ordinary weekends, any of which can be turned into something special by sharing them with people you care about.

The best parties, large or small, are those that have a theme. Take your cues from the seasons and holidays, or from the types of food you're serving. You might even consider celebrating a nonoccasion, like having an "unbirthday party." Here are some party theme ideas:

- All holidays, but the lesser-known ones are particularly fun: Bastille Day, May Day, Cinco de Mayo, etc. Research those that have some connection with your heritage.
- Entertaining in conjunction with special events in which you and your friends are participating: horse shows, dog shows, charity benefits, boating, racing, or local sporting events.
- Entertaining around events you're *not* attending: Derby Day, the Indy 500, the U.S. Open, the World Series, etc. You can always watch it on TV.
- Seasonal motifs: a rose garden, fall harvest, Jack Frost, etc.
- Themes directly related to the menu: Chinese, Italian, Mexican, Greek, etc.
- Events related to someone's good fortune: bon voyage, welcome home, job promotion, etc.
- Design motifs: Art Deco, Victorian, Baroque, etc.

There are all sorts of ways to create and sustain a party motif. Be imaginative. Use toys, game pieces, colored paper, pots, plants, figurines, and other things you have around the house, or things you make yourself. Check out the local dime store or crafts shop for ideas. Also, don't dismiss the idea of party favors at each place or parting "gifts" for your guests. Adults love surprises as much as children do, although they may not want to admit it.

Hospitality Tips

If you've ever eaten in a truly fine restaurant, you know that presentation is intrinsic to the pleasure of the dining experience. Luscious food properly showcased tempts the eye as well as the palate, while also indicating the pride and generous hospitality of the host.

Anytime you have guests in your home, even for informal occasions, you'll want to be sure that your dining table or buffet areas are artfully decorated and arranged. The tabletop doesn't have to be super fancy to show you care, but it should be conveniently set and color coordinated. (By the way, this goes for everyday meals for the two of you, too.)

Ambience and a feeling of hospitality extend beyond the dining room, however. When you entertain, you'll want your whole house to reflect a party mood. Candles on coffee tables or sideboards, arrangements of fresh flowers in the foyer, guest soaps in the bath, and other thoughtful touches all say "Welcome, we're glad you came." These and the following little extras are appreciated by your guests:

- Keep fresh flowers in your home, particularly during the winter. A small bouquet each week won't break the bank, but will do wonders to lift the spirits.
- Take a cue from fine hotels and keep a basket with miniature soap, hand lotion, perfume, shampoo, etc. on your bathroom vanity. Visitors, especially those staying overnight, will appreciate it.
- If you often have out-of-town houseguests, make up a "hospitality packet" that includes a city map, sightseeing guide, postcards, even bus or subway tokens. The packet shows them you care and makes a nice memento of their visit.
- Don't forget the music. Whether it's salsa for a South American supper or soft rock as a background for quiet conversation, nothing sets a mood like music. And please turn off the television when company arrives!

Keeping Records

Well-known hostesses have social secretaries who help them keep track of who's been invited to what, what was served, and how everything went. Not only do such records provide an evaluation of the party, they also insure that menus and guest combinations are not repeated when the same groups of people are entertained regularly.

As newlyweds, you probably don't entertain enough yet to need a social secretary, but there are lots of years and parties ahead. Records of what you've served and how it was received, including the cost and preparation time, can be invaluable in building a repertoire of reliable, adaptable menus you can count on over and over again.

You can buy books for this task, usually where cookbooks are sold, or you can make your own entertaining notebook using the following sample sheet as a guide. You could also adapt this form for use in a database software program in your home computer.

Home Entertaining Record

Date: _____   Occasion: _____

Theme: _____   Decorations: _____

Guests:

_____   _____

_____   _____

_____   _____

_____   _____

Menu: Recipe Book/Page:

_____   _____

_____   _____

_____   _____

_____   _____

_____   _____

Accompanying Beverages:

_____   _____   _____

_____   _____   _____

Approximate   Average
Total Cost: _____ Number _____ = Cost per Person _____

Notes on Preparation: _____

_____

_____

_____

Comments: _____

_____

CHAPTER 4
Dealing with In-Laws

*T*here's an old adage about sons and daughters; perhaps you've heard it:

> A son is a son till he takes a wife,
> A daughter is a daughter for the rest of her life.

Not! At least, better not. Realistically speaking, you are always a son and always a daughter, and you will always have responsibilities in those roles. But the choice of who comes first in your life is made, and made publicly, on your wedding day. From then on, no one else, not your parents nor any other family member, can ever be put ahead of your spouse—ever. It may sound cruel, ungrateful even, but that's the way it has to be. Otherwise, the marriage bond will never be secure.

This concept of leaving the family and "cleaving" to the new spouse gives a lot of people trouble, especially in the beginning. First of all, newlyweds aren't always sure how to define "putting someone first" and don't always recognize when it's appropriate, and necessary, to take a stand. For instance, does asking your husband to ride the bus home so you can have the car to visit your sister in the hospital mean that you're putting her first? Then again, is your husband being selfish, or manipulative, if he sees it that way?

And then there are the families, especially close ones, who find it hard to relinquish their role as primary support giver and who may actually fear what they see as a growing physical and psychological distance resulting from your marriage. Even well-meaning in-laws can become smothering and controlling in their desire to preserve and protect their relationship with their own children. "We're not losing a daughter, we're gaining a son," they say. Yeah, right.

All in all, it's a pretty complicated business because, for better or worse, you're stuck with the family you have and, for better or worse, they've made you who you are. And now, for better or worse, you've also taken on someone else's family. So, dealing with in-laws, your own and each other's, becomes one of the major, and sometimes most difficult, adjustments newlyweds have to make.

The good news, though, is that most couples manage to preserve meaningful relationships with their own families, while also successfully forging new bonds with their in-laws. Various surveys and studies conducted on family ties repeatedly show that, in spite of changing lifestyles, long-distance relocations, and other demands of life, most Americans continue to report strong kinship ties and to iden-

---

ᠭᢒ᠍᠍ᢗ᠍ᢲ   *DO YOU SEE YOURSELF HERE?*   ᠭᢒ᠍᠍ᢗ᠍ᢲ

- Have unexpected conflicts erupted between your spouse and his or her family?
- Are you becoming aware of patterns of behavior in either of you or your families that you did not notice before the marriage?
- Are you feeling unsure of your role in your spouse's family conflicts?
- Does either of you have unresolved issues from childhood with your families, siblings, or other relatives?
- Do you feel that your spouse is not sufficiently separated from his or her family?
- Do you feel your spouse is trying to shift some of the emotional burden for his or her family onto you?
- Are you living with your in-laws or contemplating doing so?
- Are differences in family backgrounds, religion, race, or culture presenting on-going problems between you and your families?
- Do the two of you argue because of your families?

Once again, "yes" answers mean you need to read on.

---

tify relationships with immediate and extended family members as a primary source of personal satisfaction and support (Chadwick & Heaton, 169–70).

Family life is important, and it's worth devoting at least as much time and attention to cementing relationships with your in-laws as it is with your friends and coworkers. The groundwork, and the ground rules, you lay as newlyweds will become a foundation for life.

Understanding Family Patterns

Marriage is a bonding process. Two people, unrelated biologically, make a physical, mental, and emotional commitment to each other in a state of what is commonly called "love." The two people alone, or with any children that result from their union, constitute a new family. It follows, then, that one who has managed to maintain a "free but connected relationship" (in other words, a healthy relationship) with his or her parent family will be better able to achieve such an ideal in his or her own family. For most people, the home life before marriage is the only preparation and role model for establishing their own future families.

Besides the blending of two personalities in marriage, the newly formed family is also a composite of the two from which the spouses came. Certain values, attitudes, and traditions may have their roots several generations back on either side. So, the reality is that we marry not only a spouse *and* his or her parents, but the whole family tree. Whatever conflicts are yet unresolved in that family will, inevitably, encroach upon the new marital relationship.

Understanding family systems and genealogies helps us understand ourselves and others. The whole family, taken as a unit with aunts, uncles, cousins, grandparents, and everyone else, projects a singular approach to certain life issues. You could say that the clan has a collective personality, and aspects of that inherited personality are brought by each member into the new marriages.

- Why does a family celebrate weddings or anniversaries in a specific way?
- How does it handle money or household responsibilities? How does it mourn or face a crisis?
- What are the collective attitudes toward sex, religion, politics?
- Most importantly, whether the family in question is your own or your spouse's, how do you accept or reject these attitudes and values?

Practically speaking, you two have to consider how easy is it going to be to avoid inherited beliefs and behaviors that are undesirable in your own marriage and family. In order to fully understand your families' dynamics, you have to ask these kinds of questions.

Beyond the drama of the collective cast of characters, each family member also plays a specific role. You know the types: there are good kids and bad kids, the rebel, the favorite, the martyr, the mediator, the responsible one, and on and on. The family system, as it has been operating since childhood, depends on the complicity of the players in these designated roles, and so the roles easily extend into adulthood, at least within the family of origin.

How do those roles affect your marriage? In as many ways as there are roles. For instance, if you marry the "family problem solver," then you can expect phone calls and requests for advice and assistance from your in-laws for as long as your spouse continues to play that role, which may be forever. If you married the "favorite son," it may take you a long time to prove that you're good enough to be his wife—and you may never prove it. If you married "the troublemaker," you will be forever trying to explain, to make excuses, and to smooth things over. And so it goes. . . . The same goes for you and your role in your own family, too. Inevitably, your spouse will be affected by the part you play.

Understanding the family systems, and the roles each of you plays in those systems, can be enormously helpful in explaining the behaviors of other family members toward you and in maintaining your objectivity about family matters. The actions of other family members and the stories they tell about the past can also help you better understand your spouse. The recognition of family patterns, both collective and individual, provides a valuable source of self-knowledge and a reasonable gauge of behavior in other situations. At best, they can help you develop happy, successful relationships between you and both your families; at the very least, they can help you recognize negative traits and unresolved conflicts so you can learn to overcome them.

(Note: We have been talking about typical roles and patterns of behavior in normal families, not destructive roles or abusive behaviors in dysfunctional families. If either of you feels that your role in your family has harmed you or that negative family traits threaten your happiness together, then you should consider professional counseling to help you recognize and change those detrimental patterns.)

Draw a Family Picture

As we've been discussing, people don't exist in a vacuum; each of us is part of several larger systems of interdependent relationships, the most important one being the family. What happens to one person in the system usually reverberates to affect everyone else.

Family pictures, called "genograms," are visual representations of family histories, sort of a behavioral/psychological genealogy chart. They are generally associated with Dr. Murray Bowen's Family Systems Theory, and are widely used today by family therapists (McGoldrick & Gerson, 5). Because genograms depict significant events and information at a glance, they can help family members see themselves from a broader, more objective perspective.

For clinical purposes, genograms can get very complicated and can require considerable skill on the part of a therapist to construct and interpret. But you can create a simple version, for knowledge and fun, much in the same way that one researches genealogy. In fact, if you have a family genealogy chart already, that provides an ideal foundation for this project. Otherwise, you'll have to search your memory and your records, and perhaps interview some relatives for pertinent information.

Begin with a blank chart that looks something like Figure 4.

Instructions

Use circles for women and squares for men, and always work from left to right, that is, husbands on left, oldest siblings from left. Connect married partners with a line, and dangle children of that union from the line. Include names, birth dates, death dates, and marriage dates. (Try to be as accurate as possible with dates, otherwise, approximate as best you can.) Then, in addition, include as much of the following information as you have:

health problems/causes of death
professions/talents
education
achievements/awards
weaknesses/failures
divorce/widowhood/remarriage
stepchildren, adopted children, twins
birth order (left to right)
religion
nationality
major life events: immigration, religious conversion, accidents, etc.
important dates or other significant events
include any significant, though nonrelated, extended family members, such as
    housekeepers, godparents, or others, in the chart, too
indicate, by circling or highlighting, the dominant partner in each marriage

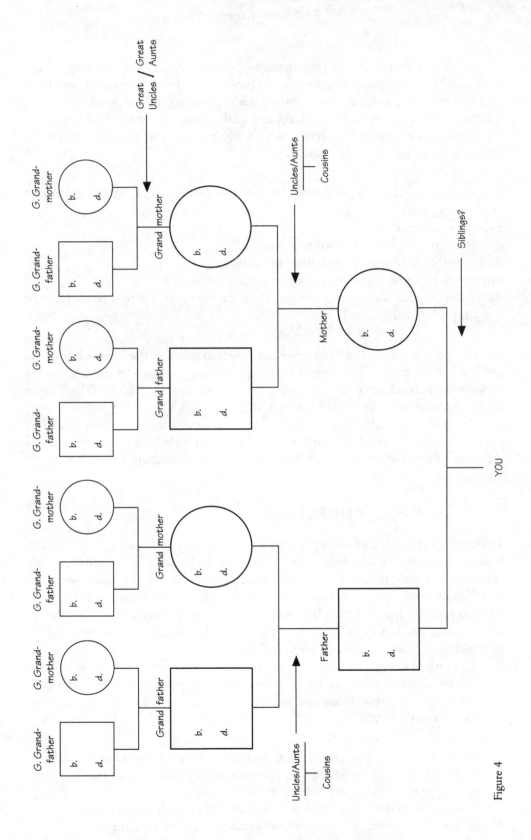

Figure 4

69

If yours is a large family with many important events, you may have to use additional sheets of paper to construct a chronology of those events. There is no one way to do a genogram, even among the experts, so you can code and cross-reference however you wish. As long as it makes sense to you, it will work.

You'll each need to do your own family picture and then analyze it for repetitive patterns. You may find

repeated significance of the same calendar date or month on which important
   events occur
marriage patterns
dominant traits, professions, or talents
dominant problems, such as alcohol or addiction
migratory patterns, job changes, or major life upheavals
deviation or rebellion from patterns, such as marrying outside one's faith or
   adopting an alternate lifestyle

When you have each analyzed your own genogram, put the two side by side and look at them together. Coincidence or prophecy? What patterns do you see in your own family that are also reflected in your spouse's chart? What might that tell you about why you chose each other?

Good traits or bad, awareness is the key to avoiding those behaviors you don't want to repeat. Examining your family pictures can only lead to a better understanding of yourself and each other, and better communication between you.

Separation Anxieties

Evaluating one's self and one's place in a family is not always easy, and differentiating ourselves from the roles we play can be even harder. Our families provide for our most basic needs of love and acceptance and, as we get older, we try to fulfill their needs and expectations of us in return. At some point, though, we have to separate from our families and establish our independence—intellectually, socially, and emotionally. Psychologists call this process "separation and individuation," and it marks an individual's maturity.

The task of separation is one we all face to become our own person, and the role we continue to play as an adult in the family is a good indicator of just how successful this separation/maturation process has been. Each of you needs to assess that for yourselves:

* What are your real or implied responsibilities to your family of origin?
* What are the ways in which you continue to depend on your family: financial support, decision making, emotional support?
* What is the nature of your personal relationship with your parents?
* What is the nature of your personal relationships with siblings?
* How have these relationships contributed to your self-esteem? Do they continue to affect your self-image?

People marrying later and having been on their own longer would seem to be positive signs of the maturity of today's newlyweds. Yet, age and career success can be misleading. Someone can be physically and economically independent while still being emotionally attached.

Jane and Bob were both fast-track career professionals when they met and fell in love. The only difference was that Jane was living and working in the city of her birth, whereas Bob had already moved several times. The couple was not surprised when Bob was transferred again right after their wedding, but Jane was surprised at how difficult the adjustment to the move became for her.

"We found a great apartment, I learned my way around, and I even landed a good job," she says. "The only problem was that my parents and my sisters were clear across the country. I never realized before moving so far away what that would mean. I couldn't just pick up the phone and chat for an hour, or run by to borrow a scarf or a handbag, or go to the movies with one of them when Bob was working late. We weren't even together for Thanksgiving that first year! It was awful. I missed them so much."

Bob and Jane still live clear across the country from her family and she still misses their close proximity, but she's adjusting. "I'm trying to make do with fewer phone calls and more letters, and visits home twice a year. And I'm buying all my own accessories now!" she laughs. "It's still difficult, though, especially on holidays. I know intellectually that closeness doesn't really depend on geography, but having said that, I also know that I have transferred some of my emotional needs from my family to Bob. Come to think of it, maybe that's a good thing."

It's not only a good thing, it's absolutely necessary because that kind of mutual reliance and primary trust must be vested in each other before a couple can really become a couple. Interestingly, some newlyweds achieve this easily, perhaps having already begun to unify and to assert their couplehood while engaged; for others, like Jane, a redirected reliance on the new spouse may literally require a physical relocation away from family members.

Loosening Family Ties

The more directly involved family members have been in your life—through lending money, giving advice, or helping out with routine chores—the harder it is to let go of that presence and to turn, instead, to your spouse. That doesn't mean, of course, that the support of family is no longer necessary, but simply that you and your spouse are each other's primary caregivers now. You must rely on each other first and foremost.

A certain amount of "separation anxiety" is to be expected, especially in close families, while this redirection takes place, and parents and siblings will feel some of the anxiety and awkwardness, too. After all, they have to come to terms with the fact that they are in second place now, and that is never easy. In their attempts to stay connected and extend their closeness to a new son or daughter-in-law, they may seem meddlesome and interfering. Or, they may go the other way in their attempt to respect your new status and privacy; that is, their calls and visits may become so infrequent that you wonder if everyone has died!

Even families that weren't all that close before may feel an intensified loss at the marriage of one of their children and may begin to behave in surprising ways. One newlywed tells how her mother complained that the couple never came to dinner *anymore*. "And I said, 'No Ma. It's not *anymore*. We never came to your house for dinner period, because you don't cook. I didn't come for dinner when I was single either, so what on earth are you talking about?'"

Families are people, and they're not perfect. They forget, or they want to remember things differently, or they want your marriage to be a new beginning for them, too. Be patient. In time, the estrangement and awkwardness you might feel now in family situations will ease and more relaxed ways of relating to each other will return.

Setting Precedents

In the first chapter, we talked about setting precedents for behaviors between you that, once established, would be almost impossible to change. Well, that advice times ten goes for setting precedents within families.

"At first, you know, I thought she was just trying to be helpful," says Rose of her mother-in-law who used to drop by her house in the afternoons while Rose was at work. "I mean, she'd always do little things, the dishes or laundry, and she'd leave me notes. But then, after the baby came and I was home, I didn't appreciate her dropping in unannounced anymore. She'd come in and try to take over and tell me what to do and how to do it, and I just didn't need that."

The more Rose thought about it, the more she decided that she didn't need her mother-in-law to have a key to her house either—a key that her husband had given his mother without Rose's knowledge because he just "didn't want to get into it with Mom." So Rose played the heavy; she insisted that her mother-in-law call before visiting in the future, and she secured the return of the house key. Now the two women barely speak.

"It's awkward when your mother-in-law doesn't speak to you, but that really isn't the worst of it," Rose says. "The worst part is that this situation has brought something to light between my husband and me: I realize that he has always dealt with his mother by not dealing with her. Now that I'm unable to deal with her for him, he seems to resent me for it. Is he going to get to the point where he doesn't deal with me either?"

What Other Couples Say . . .

When couples argue over their in-laws, it is generally because one spouse feels the other is being manipulated by his or her parents or siblings. Family interference is almost always blamed on the inability, or the unwillingness, of one's spouse to handle his or her own relatives with firmness, fairness, and objectivity.

Good question, several questions really, and all emanating from precedents innocently set. Why didn't Rose say something early on about her mother-in-law invading the privacy of her home? Why didn't she take a stand when her husband gave away a house key without her knowledge or permission? And why didn't she see how emotionally distant her husband's relationship with his mother really was, and recognize it as a pattern that could be projected onto her?

Why? Perhaps because newlyweds want to keep the peace and avoid conflict as long as they can (which could also be a dangerous precedent to set in a relationship). More than likely, though, it was because neither Rose nor her husband could see the complex issues at stake in such an apparently innocent situation.

Dr. Paul Dasher, a New Jersey psychologist who specializes in pre- and postmarital counseling, says that people come to marriage with all sorts of baggage, mostly repressed childhood issues that don't surface until well after the wedding. "There may be some clues that there are problems and strained relationships," he says, "but everyone chalks it all up to prewedding stress and they try to dispel any doubts or conflicts. They may do that for a while after marriage, too. Typically, couples only seek help and clarification when things finally explode."

Dr. Dasher points out that a strong case could be made for educating one's self about psychological issues before marriage, and for using counseling as a preventative rather than a curative measure. Then, couples might be better able to recognize what the real issues are and to avoid setting dangerous precedents, both between themselves and within their families.

"The ability to evaluate one's self critically, and to absorb loving criticism from the significant other is the most important skill in marriage," he says. "That skill is absolutely essential for avoiding the biggest killer in marriage—the intrusion of repressed childhood issues and lingering emotional problems from before the marriage." In other words, Rose's husband has to get a handle on his relationship with his mother.

One of the most common, and most cumbersome, precedents all too easily set in marriage is the ready transference of a man's social and emotional responsibilities, particularly those for his family, to his wife. Suddenly, she's supposed to buy all the gifts, remember all the birthdays and anniversaries, make all the phone calls, issue all the invitations, *and* deal with his mother. Why? Is a son really only a son until he takes a wife? Think about it.

Many other common family precedents are set early on in marriage, including rigid expectations regarding the celebration of holidays ("Christmas Eve is *always* at Martha's house"), jobs that are traditionally performed by a particular family member ("Uncle Marvin does *everybody's* taxes"), or tastes and habits that must be continued (*"All* of the children and their families spend part of the summer at the beach house"). None of these precedents are a big deal unless you agree unwittingly and then grow to resent it. Then they can cause serious conflict. You don't have to question everything or "buck the system" at every turn to achieve sufficient separation and independence from your families. But, it is wise to discuss the expectations each of your families has of you as a couple, and to make sure you're both aware of the ramifications that expectations honored today will have for tomorrow. Whether it's your family or his, the two of you will have to stand solidly together on whatever positions you take. And that precedent of solidarity as a couple has to be set from the beginning if it is ever to be taken seriously later on.

Mothers-in-Law: No Joke

After decades of reinforcement by stand-up comics and television sitcoms, the meddlesome mother-in-law has become such a cliché that people are sometimes reluctant to admit that they actually have a good relationship with a mother-in-law—even, heaven forbid, like her! But it does happen, quite often in fact.

A 1987 National Survey of Families and Households found that the vast majority of men and women, approximately 75 percent, rated their relationships with their mothers-in-law at the high end (5, 6, or 7) of a seven-point scale. Believe it or not, these same respondents rated their relationship with their mothers-in-law even slightly higher (by one or two percentage points) than with their fathers-in-law (Chadwick & Heaton, 81). Incidentally, and perhaps not surprisingly, the older the respondents, the better the relationships with in-laws in general.

Most discussions about the mother-in-law focus on the particular nature of her relationship with a daughter-in-law, on preemptive claims of affection and territorial rights. Let's face it: when a man chooses a wife, she becomes the primary woman in his life, and his mother knows it. That's the way it has to be, of course, but that doesn't mean it doesn't hurt a little, or take some getting used to.

If the mother-son relationship has been a close one, then there's bound to be a tinge of jealousy at having been demoted in the hierarchy of his affections. The slightest thing can serve to remind Mom that she's been replaced: a belated birthday card or a forgotten phone call. If the mother-son relationship has been less than close, or even distant, the man's obvious affection for his new wife can engender resentment, especially if he also spends time with his wife's mother and seems to enjoy the company of her family.

It is true that husbands tend to be more easily absorbed into their wives' family network and to spend more time with her side of the family. It's not deliberate; it's probably just that daughters show closeness to their own families by being physically as well as emotionally close. And, since the female partner usually makes most social arrangements, wives, especially newlywed wives, are much more likely to make social plans with their own family members. Whatever the reason, though, his mother, who is already feeling sensitive about her new place in her son's life, can feel doubly rejected and replaced.

The awkwardness between mother-in-law and daughter-in-law is not one-sided, however; jealousies and sensitivities can work the other way, too. A new wife often feels threatened by her husband's closeness to his mother, or feels that she has to compete with her way of doing things—her cooking, her house-keeping, her knowledge and efficiency. The newlywed, insecure about her own strengths and still settling into an unfamiliar role, can easily misinterpret her mother-in-law's well-intentioned gestures.

Sometimes, of course, there are simply personality conflicts. Just as all of our good friends aren't necessarily fond of each other, isn't it unreasonable also to expect that family members who share the love of one person will automatically love each other? It just isn't realistic.

As the newest members of each other's families, you two have a special obligation to be sensitive, even conciliatory, if for no other reason than you're younger and more adaptable. You don't have to love your mother-in-law or fa-ther-in-law, but they do deserve respect. Think about it this way: these are the people who created the person you love most in the world.

Sibling Rivalries

Much has been written about sibling relationships among children, but interest in adult sibling relationships is fairly new and not too often discussed. Only re-cently, for example, have researchers begun to examine the ways in which piv-otal life events, such as getting married, can alter the nature of adult sibling re-lationships.

In an article about adult sibling rivalry in *Psychology Today,* writer Jane Mersky Leder found in background interviews that stories of strained rela-tionships immediately following the marriage of a brother or sister far out-weighed stories of marriages that enhanced sibling connections. Often, bad sibling relationships got worse, and even good relationships became strained. Why is that?

Part of the reason may be that growing up with siblings, giving and taking, sharing and fighting, in many ways approximates a future marital relationship. Brothers and sisters are intimately connected, and those early bonds and pat-terns of behavior, positive or negative, persist into adulthood. It's the old "fam-ily systems" theory at work again.

Siblings who are very close as adults, who run around together or maybe even live together, are displaced, much as close friends are, when the brother or sister takes a spouse. If that new spouse is very different or doesn't fit into the family very well, a strain on the sibling relationship is inevitable and resentments are bound to occur.

Less than perfect relationships, including adult sibling rivalries, can also be intensified with the marriage of a brother or sister. Often, the new spouse will adopt the same posture and position as the sibling toward the brother- or sister-in-law; that is, the spouses of siblings will become competitive or jealous or ma-nipulative of the affections of others in the family. Who makes more money? Who will inherit? Who has brighter children?

At the extreme, of course, such conflicts indicate deep-seated problems and dysfunctional relationships, but even "normal" rivalries can escalate to dangerous levels if you let them. "It's hard not to get drawn into a competitive situation, especially when everyone else in the family accepts that as the norm," says one newlywed whose husband is in business with his brother.

"I'm told that the two boys competed for everything their whole lives—in school, in sports, in love—and that it's just the nature of their relationship. So now it's a contest of who brings in the bigger accounts or who works longer hours. I don't like it. I don't like what this so-called 'good-natured competition' brings out in my husband, and I don't like the way my sister-in-law gets into the act either."

Obviously, this newlywed is either going to have to learn to totally ignore the situation or to enlist her husband's help in finding ways for her to avoid the "good-natured fun" the others seem to enjoy. Either way, she will have to resolve the issue of her husband's sibling rivalry before it begins to affect their marriage and family relationships.

Sibling Intrusions

Just as marriage affects sibling relationships, the siblings can also affect the marriage. The dependent sibling who demands constant help and support can strain the resources, and the patience, of a new spouse; the irresponsible sibling who constantly shifts his share of family burdens onto someone else may become even more irresponsible when a new spouse is available to help carry the load. Even the perfect sibling relationship can lead to unfair comparisons and expectations of a new spouse.

The latter is especially true of twins. "Mark and Bill are identical. They act alike, think alike, look alike," says Mark's wife. "They have always gotten along extremely well because they are mirror images of each other. Of course. What would they have to argue about?"

After college, Mark and Bill shared an apartment together until Bill got married. Then, Mark lived alone for a couple years until he got married.

"The initial adjustments to our day-to-day living habits were just horrendous," his wife says. "Mark simply couldn't understand why we disagreed on so many things and how I could be so different from his brother. I kept pointing out that he hadn't lived with a roommate, but with a clone. But, of course, he didn't see it that way."

Stepping in between twins may be the biggest sibling challenge of all. As Mark's and Bill's wives found out, a sympathetic sister-in-law, or brother-in-law, can be a big help because they thoroughly understand the challenge. The spouses of twins often become as close as the twins themselves, since they too are likely to share similar traits.

Marriage is a pivotal life event in sibling relationships, but the long-term effects aren't all bad. Even though reduced closeness and contact among siblings is likely after marriage, studies show that a certain stability in the relationships among brothers and sisters ensues and that most people describe those relationships in positive terms (Connidis, 980).

Living with In-Laws

Amy and Burt had it made—or so they thought. They had gone together for a long time, had a solid relationship built on equality and communication, and had even saved together for a down payment on their own condominium. The only snag in their plans occurred when they were informed that completion of their new home would be delayed by about three months.

Since their wedding date was already set, they opted to save themselves the aggravation of finding a short-term apartment lease and to accept Burt's parents' offer to move in with them for the interim. But, as is not uncommon with new constructions, bad weather, labor problems, and supply shortages turned a three-month delay into nine. By the time the couple moved into their own home, Amy questioned whether they "had any marriage left to move."

For Amy and Burt, living with in-laws was a disaster. There had been numerous arguments, hurt feelings, and things said that would be hard to forget. The couple had to recapture some of their own newlywed spirit, and they would definitely have to rebuild the relationship with Burt's parents.

More often than not, living with in-laws is a disaster. Whether it's adult children returning home or aged parents moving in, the strain of additional members being added to an existing family household is bound to be felt. For newlyweds, whose marital stability and couplehood depend on the independence they cultivate in the first year or two of their married lives, "the family nest" can be stifling.

Some couples, like Burt and Amy, don't realize the magnitude of the interpersonal challenges they face. Other couples may, for one reason or another, simply have no choice. If you find that you're one of them, or if you are contemplating such a move, the following considerations may make the situation more workable.

- **Have a family meeting.** Make sure all rights and responsibilities, financial and otherwise, are delineated and that an approximate time limit for the living arrangement is set. People can be more congenial if they know how long the situation is going to last, and if each knows what is expected of him or her within the household.
- **Respect each other's rights of privacy and ensure your own.** Adults, especially newlyweds, need space for themselves, freedom to come and go, and areas in which to entertain friends and to pursue hobbies and interests. The best arrangement is that in which common living quarters are not shared and separate entries are provided (such as the "mother-in-law suite" or two-family house).
- **Keep personal discussions and problems personal.** Not all matters between the two of you are subjects for family involvement.
- **Remember that this is not your house.** The people who own it have a right to make the rules. When you move in, you have to accept that.

Multigenerational living patterns are becoming increasingly common in America, and that's not all bad. Many couples with aged or single parents adopt such arrangements and live quite happily. As with so many other life situations, if your decision is made out of free choice, rather than from forced necessity, it is apt to have more positive results.

Dealing with Diversity

In a *New York Times* article about the newest U.S. Census information, Representative Thomas C. Sawyer, the Ohio Democrat who headed the House Census and Population Subcommittee, was quoted as saying: "The population of the United States has become much more difficult to count. . . . It is a larger, more diverse, and more mobile population than it has ever been" (Barringer, B6). Now there's an understatement! Check these facts:

- There are approximately 1 million interracial married couples, triple the number of 20 years ago (Bureau of the Census).
- More than half of all American-born Asians marry non-Asians (National Center for Health Statistics).
- The rate of interfaith marriage is almost too vast to measure.
- Of the 2.4 million marriages each year, 46 percent of them are remarriages for one or both partners (Bureau of the Census).
- There are *at least* 106 different ethnic groups in the United States (from the *Harvard Encyclopedia of American Ethnic Groups).*

And if all that diversity isn't enough to leave you dizzy, then consider the other possible variations in regional, family, and socioeconomic backgrounds, and you get a vivid picture of the nature of marriage and family in modern America. If you aren't wrestling with at least one of these differences, you are truly in the minority.

We've already discussed some of these differences and the challenges they can present in terms of newlywed adjustments, but two types of intermarriage merit special attention because they are more than just statistics. Interfaith and interracial unions present ongoing challenges to the couples and the families involved.

The Interfaith Challenge

Shirley met Vincent while she was still in high school. After the very first date, her parents forbade her to see him again because he wasn't Jewish, just as they had always discouraged any non-Jewish friendship, even with girls. But Shirley didn't listen. She saw Vincent again, and again, for seven years, all through college, but she didn't tell her parents that she was still seeing him until they got engaged.

"All hell broke loose," Shirley says. "I had to move out of my parents' house and, after all the yelling and screaming was over, we ultimately quit speaking to each other for about a year. They had visions of my marrying a Jewish doctor from Harvard and here I came with the stereotypical WASP tennis pro! There was simply no way to discuss this with them."

In contrast, Vincent's family had always been accepting of Shirley, and it was Vincent's mother who encouraged the couple to plan the wedding of their dreams, regardless of whether or not Shirley's family chose to attend. "Even so, the strain of it all definitely diminished our happiness," Shirley says.

Finally, Vincent decided to give it one last try. He went alone to Shirley's parents, explained how deeply he felt about their daughter, and made it clear that the wedding was going to take place, although everyone preferred that it be with their blessing. Amazingly, his plea worked. Both families did attend the wedding, everyone got along beautifully, and Vincent has been totally accepted ever since.

"I think my parents saw my choice as a repudiation of everything they believed in," says Shirley, "and I think my secrecy about it really made the situation worse. But, once they got to know Vincent, and once they realized that this was going to be, they simply had to come around."

Shirley and Vincent have been married a little over a year now, and they laugh about the fact that they and her parents are almost too close. "They almost want to spend too much time with us now," she says. "I think they feel guilty about the lost years."

For the time being anyway, this story has a happy ending. Even so, Shirley and Vincent admit that they never talk about having children with their families, and both express fear that problems will develop all over again whenever Shirley becomes pregnant. "I would prefer to do nothing rather than to try to raise children in both the Jewish and the Christian traditions," Vincent says, "and that's not going to go over very well with my family either." So, for now, the couple is postponing those decisions.

Avoidance won't solve the problem, of course, though a decision to have no children at all would be one way to deal with it. But, whether you're talking about the choice of spouse or future children, Shirley's identification of the fundamental problem in an interfaith marriage is right on target: the perceived repudiation of a family's most deeply held values and beliefs.

As those of you who have been through it know, even if you can get over the hurdles of planning an interfaith wedding, and even if families come to really love and accept the new spouse, questions of cultural and religious identity linger, and reassert themselves, in every philosophical discussion around the dinner table, in every holiday celebration or family rite of passage, in the future of every newborn child. That's because families persist in seeing themselves in a certain way, as identified within a certain group or tradition: Protestant, Catholic, Jewish, Muslim, or Hindu. Diluting that identification through intermarriage calls into question one of the ways a family characterizes itself, articulates its beliefs, and guarantees its continuity.

Obviously, the strains are greatest when the religion is also tied to an ethnic heritage, but frictions can also develop in less dramatically different interfaith marriages too, such as those between Protestants and Catholics, mainstream Christians and nondenominational sects, or religious fundamentalists and liberal Protestants. The more central the practice of a particular religion is in a family's

life, the more likely there are to be disagreements over specific practices and beliefs, especially where the rearing of children (grandchildren) is concerned.

There are no easy answers to these dilemmas, because religious faith is not
a matter of scientific logic and reasonable compromise. It is helpful, however, if
the two of you can make distinctions between your spiritual values and your
cultural habits. That way, while everyone else is accentuating the differences,
you two will be able to build on your similarities. Not surprisingly, those who
share a strong belief in the importance of spiritual faith find it easier to reconcile the differences in religious practice in the home.

The Interracial Challenge

"I guess the biggest problem in an interracial marriage is that your differences
are so obvious," says Audrey, who has an interracial marriage and is, herself, the
product of one. "Even when you get over the shock and resistance of your families, you still have to handle the reactions of everyone else you meet," she says.
"And people do react, no matter how sophisticated or accepting they like to
think they are. As a couple, you have to learn to deal with that, as well as with
out-and-out prejudice."

Audrey and Peter have been married for two years. She is biracial, but appears black; he is white and clearly Irish. Interestingly, both share the same religion, Catholicism, and that has eased some of the strain, at least as far as the
wedding plans and the religious training of future children were concerned.
"The fact that Peter's family are practicing Catholics and very Christian and that
my family had already been through the interracial situation made the acceptance of our decision to marry easier," Audrey says. "But there are other issues
that religion and family experience alone can't resolve."

Among the issues she cites are a persistence of negative stereotypes about
her racial group, and an insensitivity on the part of others, including her husband, to the subtle ways those negative attitudes exhibit themselves. "People
look at me and see black, not Audrey. Peter's friends do that, and some of my
in-laws still do that, but Peter doesn't understand because he doesn't think of me
as any color at all. I've had to forgive and forget a lot."

Most interracial couples do. They have to combat stereotypes and face the
issues of cultural and racial differences head on, especially with family members,
and they have to find a group of friends, usually neither all of one group or the
other, with whom they can feel comfortable and be accepted for themselves.
"And they have to be tough," Audrey says, "thick-skinned, confident in themselves, and secure in their relationship."

Celebrating Holidays

Yes, holidays are joyful, memorable, and fun, but for countless newlyweds they
are also stressful, exhausting, and fraught with conflict. For one thing, at no

other time do cultural and religious differences become such central issues as during major holidays; for another, newlyweds are the ones who are pulled between families and who spend most of the day of celebration on the road traveling from one clan to the other.

"You're damned if you do and damned if you don't," laments Geri, married two years. "We could have had everyone at our house for Easter, but no, nobody wanted to do that. It wasn't the tradition, for either family. So, this year, my husband and I decided to start our own tradition and go away for Easter. Both families had a fit. You can't win!"

No, you can't, not when you're young and newly married, and certainly not when you're childless and have no excuse for not "schlepping." Younger couples spend the first few years trying to find their place within existing family traditions, trying to establish some holiday traditions of their own, and trying to negotiate and accommodate two sets of family demands.

Some holidays are worse than others. Thanksgiving, for instance, is very difficult for Jewish couples, because Hanukkah is not a major celebration and Christmas is nonexistent. So, Thanksgiving becomes the only fall/winter family holiday. Spending it with one family means you can't spend it with the other.

Holiday arrangements may be less complicated when only one family lives nearby, but then their expectations can be more rigid, too. "For three years now I've wanted to spend Thanksgiving Day in the City at the Macy's Parade," says a young man who is not originally from the New York area, "but my wife's family just won't hear of it. Every year we have a row over it, and every year I give in, but I'm not giving up."

It's very difficult to modify existing traditions within a family or to assert your right to create your own, but sometimes you have to. That's especially true for interfaith/intercultural couples who must find ways to honor, respect, and integrate the customs and rituals that are important to each of them. Sure, you can spend Passover with one family and Easter with the other, but what about traditions in your own home, and what about the future with your children?

Caring Solutions

A priest and a rabbi in the San Francisco Bay area have started The Interfaith Community to help couples and families learn how to blend traditions and celebrate together. (See Appendix for resource.) "Our only agenda is inclusiveness," says Rabbi Charles Familant. "We alter traditional celebrations and rituals so that everyone can participate and no one is simply watching from the outside."

The participants do all the work, plan the services and the ceremonies, and educate themselves in the process. The Community might have a seder on Good Friday, or a December celebration combining the lighting of an Advent wreath and a menorah. The 200-member community includes Catholic, Protestant, Jewish, and Buddhist traditions right now, but the group is evolving and expanding and hopes to get clergy from other denominations involved. "It's very exciting and enriching for all of us," says Rabbi Familant.

Ideally, that's the way holiday celebrations ought to be for everybody. Do what you can to make that true for you and your families. Here are some ideas:

- Decorate the dinner table even if it's just for the two of you. Use paper napkins with the appropriate holiday motif for drinks, snacks, or dessert.
- Celebrate the seasons and create little traditions of your own. Go pick strawberries or blueberries in the summer and then spend the day baking pies or making jam together. Make seasonal decorations for your front door. Chop down your Christmas tree at a tree farm. Force bulbs indoors so you'll have daffodils and tulips for spring.
- Greeting cards aren't reserved just for Christmas. Cards and notes sent for other holidays during the year make those you love part of your celebration, particularly when they live far away.
- If you are in an interfaith/intercultural marriage, study up. Read and learn all you can about the history of each other's traditions so you will understand and appreciate the rituals and ceremonies of holiday celebrations.
- Invite your families to your house for some holiday they usually don't celebrate, such as Valentine's Day or St. Patrick's Day, or even Arbor Day! Who knows. You may start a tradition of your own.
- Remember how hard precedents are to break. If you're going to deviate from some traditional family celebration, better to do it early on.

Forget Me Not

Aunts, uncles, nieces, nephews, cousins—so many people to get to know and remember, especially if your families are large. Trying to keep up with important dates can be a real challenge, particularly when you're still trying to match the names with the faces.

Use the handy "Forget Me Not" chart on the next page to make the task of endearing yourselves to your relatives more manageable.

What Other Couples Say . . .

Lots of newlyweds admit to coming away from holiday dinner tables hungry. Either they aren't accustomed to the way their in-laws cook, or they don't like the traditional foods that are served.

What do you do if you don't eat Christmas goose or Thanksgiving turkey? "You eat before you leave home," says one newlywed who's a vegetarian.

Forget Me Not

January

Day	Name	Relation	B'day A'sry	Card	Gift

February

Day	Name	Relation	B'day A'sry	Card	Gift

March

Day	Name	Relation	B'day A'sry	Card	Gift

April

Day	Name	Relation	B'day A'sry	Card	Gift

May

Day	Name	Relation	B'day A'sry	Card	Gift

June

Day	Name	Relation	B'day A'sry	Card	Gift

July

Day	Name	Relation	B'day A'sry	Card	Gift

August

Day	Name	Relation	B'day A'sry	Card	Gift

September

Day	Name	Relation	B'day A'sry	Card	Gift

October

Day	Name	Relation	B'day A'sry	Card	Gift

November

Day	Name	Relation	B'day A'sry	Card	Gift

December

Day	Name	Relation	B'day A'sry	Card	Gift

CHAPTER 5
Cultivating Intimacy

P oets and philosophers have been pondering the mysteries of love for centuries, but in late twentieth-century America, scientists have taken the lead. Some, like Dr. John Money, a psycho-endocrinologist at the Johns Hopkins University School of Medicine, can tell us not only what happens, chemically and biologically, when two people fall in love, but also why love happens between two particular individuals. Pointing to a combination of prenatal genetic determinants and early childhood experiences, Dr. Money theorizes that each of us has in mind a "developmental template" of the ideal lover and love affair. He calls this a "lovemap." We project this lovemap onto a real-life partner, in much the same way as meaning is projected onto a Rorschach inkblot, and that explains the powerful attraction that certain people feel for each other (Money, xv–xvi).

Perhaps, but regardless of all the scientific studies and the articles on the "chemistry" of love in the popular press, human beings are still more than their biology, and romantic love is rarely predictable. From the sublime to the ridiculous, from acts of complete and total self-sacrifice to making a complete and total fool of one's self, people will do things for love that they would never even consider doing for any other reason. The logic of those behaviors, or the lack of it, continues to confound the understanding of even the best behavioral scientists.

Thus, when you've heard what the doctors and the psychologists and, yes, even the poets have to say, you still won't have all the answers, because the inexplicable is precisely what gives human love its transcendent quality and its miraculous power. Love is what ennobles and enriches our lives, and separates us from the animals. It may even be, as the ancients thought, a matter of destiny.

Love and Sex in Marriage

Although society uses sex to sell everything from soap suds to sunny vacations, the first realization newlyweds make about sex in marriage is that it is inextricably linked to the nature of their love and the day-to-day fluctuations in their relationship. As Thomas W. Roberts, Ph.D., states in the *Journal of Marital and Family Therapy,* "A couple's sexual response is a powerful metaphor for the overall relationship" (Roberts, 361).

﹌﹌ **DO YOU SEE YOURSELF HERE?** ﹌﹌

- Has romance, with its attendant feelings of playfulness and adventure, already begun to wane?
- Have the two of you already experienced some "cooling" of sexual desire between you?
- Are you having trouble getting your sex life in synch?
- Are you confusing sex and intimacy?
- Are past love relationships or sexual experiences clouding your present together?
- Do the two of you have different definitions of sexual morality or responsibility?
- Have jealousy and possessiveness flared between you?
- Do you feel the need for better sexual communication and/or more information about how your bodies work?
- Have there been problems with sexual hang-ups or dysfunction?
- Are you dissatisfied with the method(s) of contraception you're presently using?
- Have the two of you been unable to agree on future family planning?

"Yes" answers? Read on.

In other words, physical conditions such as illness or fatigue notwithstanding, the quality of your sex life is a fairly reliable barometer of how things are going between you in general. When you're feeling good about yourself and happy with your mate, sexual expression is likely to be more playful and adventurous. Likewise, if you're perturbed with each other, you're less apt to feel amorous. Marriage counselors commonly find that couples who are really estranged don't even face each other when they sleep, much less touch or make love.

Sexual desire and gratification bring an added dimension, and sometimes an added pressure, to the marital bond. But, the freedom to express one's self sexually in an atmosphere of complete trust and security is also one of the most universally cited pleasures of married life. To the extent that a satisfying sexual relationship grows out of the security and trust between you, self-esteem and self-worth are increased in direct proportion. Furthermore, knowing you are loved, totally and completely, from the tops of your temples to the tips of your toes, makes facing some of life's other difficulties a whole lot easier.

Sex may, indeed, be a metaphor in marriage, but let's not forget that it can also be separated from love and become a powerful tool in its own right. It can be used to soothe and sustain, or to hurt and punish; it can be calm and comforting, or torrid and passionate; it can be teasing and romantic, or routine and mechanical. And it can be all of those things at one time or another for the same couple!

Great sex alone will not be able to save a marriage when it has nothing else going for it, but it can certainly make a good marriage even stronger and happier. Like all other forms of couple communication, sexual communication is built through trust and understanding and deepens with time and experience. As you learn to read each other's unspoken sexual messages, as well as to listen to the messages that are explicitly expressed, you will become better lovers. And that will make for a better marriage and a happier you.

Cooling It!

One of the most upsetting revelations newlyweds uncover about human nature is how fast passion wanes when the object of one's desire is freely available and fully accessible.

"We had a long-distance courtship for over two years," says Holly, "so the buildup of romantic anticipation and sexual desire was incredible. Honestly, when we first got married and were with each other all the time, the sex was amazing, truly amazing, all consuming in fact. We sometimes forgot to eat. I had trouble getting to work on time. It was ridiculous." She laughs.

But then . . . "I don't know. His studies, my job, money problems." Holly pauses to think about it. "I mean, it couldn't go on like that forever, because we'd never get anything else done, you know. But it was a shock to wake up one day eight or nine months into the marriage and realize that two weeks had gone by without our making love. I felt like one of those cases in the women's magazines, and all I could think of was what would it be like in 20 years if this was happening already?"

The declining frequency of sexual intercourse is the most disturbing, most universally talked about concern of early married life. It doesn't happen as rapidly for couples who haven't slept together before marriage, but it still happens, to everybody, and everybody thinks it's abnormal when it does.

"Two people must get past the lust and obsession stage of sexual intimacy in order for a relationship to grow," says Dr. Judy Seifer, sex therapist and president of the American Association of Sex Educators, Counselors and Therapists. "Couples see the waning of sexual excitement as a negative, but actually, it is a positive sign, an indication that the relationship is moving to a different, deeper level. That only happens when couples have complete confidence in the availability and fidelity of each other."

At this stage, "availability" comes to mean being available in other ways: closeness, caring affection, respect, and friendship. And, curiously, while frequency may diminish somewhat, the intensity of the sexual act will be heightened. The more confident and committed two people feel in their relationship, the more selfless and giving they will be in their sexual responses. This is not just sex; this is making love, an act in which the physical, emotional, intellectual, and spiritual dimensions of the partnership converge.

From Sex to Intimacy

"One of the myths that persists in our society is that if two people are in love, they'll just do what comes naturally, and a satisfying, intimate sexual relationship will just happen," says Dr. Seifer. "That may get you pregnant, but that won't get you satisfaction. Nor will it deepen the sexual intimacy between you."

The other myth that persists, despite feminist objections to the contrary, is that men are supposed to know how to please a woman sexually, and that women are supposed to be coy and deferential, especially in matters of sex. These attitudes emanate directly from the double standard still at work in our society (the one that says boys will be boys, so it's natural for them to prove their masculinity through experience, but "nice girls" are sexual "gatekeepers" and are not supposed to be open, much less knowledgeable, about their sexual needs).

Mixed messages like these work subliminally to ingrain Puritan attitudes and foster sexual inhibitions, even among intelligent people who should know better. "The truth is that most couples find it infinitely more comfortable to engage in sex than to talk about it, even when that performance is repeatedly unsatisfying," says Dr. Seifer.

The rhythms and patterns of complex sexual responses can be stubbornly uncooperative at first, even for couples who are seemingly comfortable with each other and who are sincerely trying to please. It takes practice, but it also takes talking openly about sexual needs and desires. Regardless of how "knowledgeable or experienced" they are, couples have to work together to become super lovers and to become sensitive to the sensual/erotic nuances between them.

Every person, every partner, is different, so that even if you and/or your mate had sexual experience with other partners before the marriage, that does not mean that the sexual synchronization between the two of you will happen automatically. Furthermore, you simply cannot separate the sexual from the emotional and the psychological in marriage; satisfying sex can only exist in a climate of complete and total trust. As feelings of mutual trust and security increase between you, so will the passion and power of your lovemaking.

That kind of sexual synchronization can be one of the biggest challenges newlyweds face, and achieving it takes practice, patience, and sensitivity. If you two waited until you were married to have sexual intercourse, you will have to be patient and understanding, even in the midst of your new sexual excitement, as you learn more about yourself and how to respond to each other. You can't expect to dismiss all the cultural myths and set aside all the learned inhibitions of your courtship days overnight.

On the other hand, if you two were involved with each other sexually before the marriage, then you have probably already moved past the initial stages of discovery into a more consistent, if complacent, sexual relationship. This is the next plateau, but you don't want it to become routine and predictable. Rather, you have to realize that this second plateau can be even more stimulating and exciting, and certainly more satisfying, than the first, but only if you're willing to strive toward new levels of intimacy and to guide each other in the selfless exploration of the erotic and the sensual.

The Intrusions of Life

If you can't separate sex from the emotional tenor of your relationship, you can't separate it from very real lifestyle intrusions either. Consider this candid story from a newlywed, a resident in a big city hospital:

What Other Couples Say . . .

Husbands admit to being disappointed, but not really surprised, to find that sexual frequency diminishes rather rapidly after the honeymoon as the responsibilities of life intrude. Some will even go so far as to also admit that their lovemaking has become complacent and routine, and that their repertoire of sexual techniques doesn't seem quite as extensive as it did when they were single.

Both husbands and wives say, however, that while frequency may diminish, passion and playfulness don't have to. By making time for each other and being willing to be adventurous, couples can achieve levels of sexual satisfaction in marriage that they never dreamed were possible.

"It's like this. My wife and I are both residents, on rotation every third night. If we're lucky, we are sleeping in the same bed two nights a week. That means sex is physically impossible most of the time. When we are at home together, chances are that we are so exhausted and so mentally fatigued that any attempts at sex would be mechanical, and perfunctory, at best. That would be an insult. So, don't ask me about our sex life. We don't have one."

There is no question that the pace at which today's couples live infringes upon their time together, and their predisposition toward intimacy. Let's face it: making love takes time, sensitivity, and attentiveness, and even a certain amount of relaxation. When you're preoccupied, traveling a lot, putting in long hours, or dealing with ongoing job stress (see more in Chapter 7), the lifestyle demands are bound to affect your sex life. You are, after all, human beings, not machines.

Give yourselves a break when you are living in high-anxiety situations. Eliminate performance pressure by talking about the demands of your schedules, and forget about what other couples, or the popular press, report as normal sexual activity. Plan ahead for long, leisurely liaisons, on weekends or nights when you know you'll both be home and be rested, and see if you can't incorporate some romantic interludes, no matter how brief, into your busy days. Sex that is furtive and naughty may not be totally satisfying as a steady diet, but it can still be fun and better than nothing.

Leaving the Past Behind

"There must be at least a few 30-year-old virgins in America," Lilly sighed. "Why didn't I just let Jean-Louis think I was one of them?!"

Rationally, of course, Jean-Louis knew when he married Lilly that a 30-year-old woman had to have a past, but he didn't ask about her history and she didn't volunteer much information. Then, a couple months after the wedding, they ran into one of her former lovers, who was as charming and flirtatious as

Ten Ways to Fan the Fire of Desire

The allure of sexual adventure is a great way to keep romance alive. Here are some ideas.

1. Plant love notes in each other's lunch, or in the luggage when your spouse is traveling. Make sure the messages "sizzle" with a promise of things to come.

2. Be naughty. That is, instigate sex when the time isn't right or the situation is risky, such as just before company's due to arrive, or in the back seat of a corporate limousine.

3. Spontaneous sex is great, but prearranged "dates" for lovemaking can be fun, too. Get a bottle of your favorite wine, make a delicious dinner, and take the phone off the hook. Plan to spend uninterrupted hours making love, just as you did on your honeymoon.

4. Participate in "adult education." Get a good sex manual, or obtain a how-to sex video (see Appendix) and learn some new techniques. Then, practice, practice, practice.

5. Exercise! A University of California study found that regular exercise stimulated the libido. Other studies concur. Regular exercise also seems to make orgasm and arousal easier.

6. Buy a sexy new negligee or a provocative set of underwear. Remember: men are aroused through visual stimulation.

7. Save water; take showers together.

8. Cultivate the art of physical closeness. Hold hands, sit close, touch when you sleep. A gentle touch is a small reminder that you care.

9. Flirt with each other shamelessly in public, at a party, or while out with friends. (It'll make you the envy of every other couple present.)

10. Employ humor to play sexual games: strip poker, strip tease—use your imagination.

---

ever, at a party. The questions began and Lilly, naively, supplied more complete answers than Jean-Louis really wanted to hear.

"One thing led to another," she said. "Jean-Louis asked me about this guy, and I told him, and then he asked about others, who and when, and before I knew it I was down to defending my first kiss!"

Unfortunately, this kind of exchange is not uncommon among newly-weds because they are eager to know everything about each other and because they are full of the newfound pleasure of possession of the beloved. So, when something unexpected surfaces, curiosity is a natural impulse. Frankly, it's a deadly one.

People usually reveal secrets from the past either to assuage their own guilt, or because the so-called secrets are so inconsequential as to not be worth harboring at all. Either way, the one on the receiving end of the revelation inherits the burden of deciding what to do with it. And that can be a heavy burden, particularly when an amorous history implies inevitable comparisons to the present love.

Consider this from the recently released study by The Kinsey Institute, *Sex and Morality in the U.S.*: 60 percent of married respondents admitted that they had had *at least* one premarital sexual experience, 90 percent of them before the age of 20; about half of the responding women had premarital sex only with their future spouse, as compared to only 10 percent of the men (Klassen, Williams, & Levitt, 139–40).

There are three things worth noting from this bit of information: 1. there probably are some 30-year-old virgins out there, but not a lot of them; 2. sexual experience often starts in the teens, so that the longer one is single, the more sexual partners he or she is likely to have had; and 3. women tend to have fewer sexual partners than men, perhaps indicative of the closer association between sex and affection in the emotional makeup of women.

If your spouse was your first lover, then the past isn't as likely to be much of an issue for you, though be aware that some people can get as jealous of former loves that weren't sexually consummated as they can of those that were. (We'll talk more about jealousy later in this chapter.) But generally, a chaste history is a safe one. By the same token, if your spouse is the one with a history, do yourself a favor and don't ask for particulars. Other than the assurances you had a right to receive for health reasons before the two of you became sexually involved, don't invite comparisons by pushing for confirmation of your own superior sexual performance. The past is the past and your prior sexual history is probably not going to affect your sex life now one way or the other. You two are in the present and you two are in love; that's all that really matters.

Nobody's counseling outright dishonesty or deceit, but you each have rights to a private past. Besides, a little restraint is often much more considerate. Think about it: here you are, two newlyweds just beginning to trust each other and to feel safe and secure. Is there really anything to be gained by bringing the memory of a third party into bed with you?

Sexual Morality in Marriage

As a culture, Americans are particularly absolute and literal in their moral judgments, and nowhere more so than in issues related to sex. Look at the hottest topics of the day: homosexuality, abortion, AIDS, unwed mothers, sex education, censorship, sexual harassment. Sure, some former taboos have become more tolerated in society—divorce, cohabitation, sexually explicit books and movies—but they still are not really condoned. Public opinion polls repeatedly show that Americans continue to hold conservative attitudes on sexual morality.

At the root of all of this is the emphasis on sexual restraint inherent in a Judeo-Christian culture. Traditionally, sex was for the purpose of procreation; it was not supposed to be enjoyed, and it was certainly not supposed to be indiscriminate. To this day, sexual restraint (or denial) is somehow associated with moral superiority. In a pragmatic society, this becomes the cornerstone of middle-class morality; to flout that morality is to invite an assortment of social ills as punishment for lack of restraint: disease, loss of reputation, unwanted pregnancies, etc.

Many of the sexual taboos that become real hang-ups for couples can be traced to religious backgrounds. Moral dictates govern how we feel about everything from oral sex to artificial stimulation to birth control, and couples who don't share the same set of taboos can find themselves facing some serious moral dilemmas. Talking about the differences, of course, is the first step, but matters of individual conscience don't lend themselves easily to negotiation. It will take patience and understanding, and love, on both partners' parts to deal with these matters in a sensitive and caring way.

Then, too, couples can have dissimilar attitudes about sexual acts and preferences even when there's no religious basis for the way they feel. They just simply think something is "kinky" or weird. (Dr. Money would explain this as lovemaps that don't match.) Again, there's no arguing about the way someone feels, but discussion and patience may persuade a partner to at least try something before he or she gives it a permanent place on the list of taboos.

Making love is as much an intellectual activity as it is a physical one, so the two of you will have to think, and talk, about how you feel regarding various sexual activities. Reasonably speaking, whatever two married adults consent to in the privacy of their own home should be their business, but you don't want guilt and shame overshadowing what should be beautiful, intimate moments between you. If you can't agree, don't force the issue, at least not for the moment. Instead, accentuate the positive by concentrating on what's good in your sex life and what works to bring the greatest pleasure to you both.

Marital Fidelity

The other big moral issue in marriage is sexual fidelity, and on this one, there seems to be little divergence of opinion. Survey after survey reports that the overwhelming majority of Americans, anywhere from 70 to 90 percent of those interviewed, believe that extramarital affairs are wrong. Quite simply, most people see marriage as monogamous, even to the point of preferring serial monogamy (divorce, remarriage, divorce, remarriage) over a series of extramarital affairs.

Resisting temptation and remaining steadfast in your commitment to each other, even in rocky times, is what creating a lasting marriage is all about, and even newlyweds can be susceptible to temptation. Frankly, you're better off not to even flirt with the temptation, because once the bond of trust in your marriage is broken through a sexual indiscretion, it is hard to regain—not impossible, but hard.

An extramarital affair does not have to mean the end of the marriage, and most marriages actually do survive such affairs, provided they are isolated and short-lived. But an extramarital interlude, even just once, is an indication that there are some serious problems in the relationship, probably more serious than the two partners can handle alone. Professional intervention in the form of marital therapy is advisable, not only to save the marriage, but to help the couple rebound with a stronger, more solid relationship.

The Green-Eyed Monster

When Ted and Phyllis were first married, they worked a few blocks away from each other. Every morning, Ted and Phyllis rode the train into work together; every evening, Ted waited for Phyllis in the lobby of her building. After work, the two would either go out for a bite or to a movie, or go home together and cook. Some days, they even met for lunch. It was very romantic.

Then, about six months into the marriage, Phyllis got a promotion. Suddenly, she wasn't always available for lunch; sometimes she had early morning meetings or work to finish up before she left for the day. She and Ted didn't always ride to and from their jobs together anymore. He tried to understand, but was often lonely and resentful. Phyllis thought he was changing.

A year after their marriage, Phyllis got a *big* promotion. Now she was a full-fledged account executive, serving clients all across the country. But she also had to travel, and to entertain. Her hours were unpredictable. She tried to include Ted whenever possible, even invited him to go along on some of the business trips that took her to vacation spots, but he didn't want to be "just another line item on the expense account." He was angry and abusive whenever they were together, and he harassed her by telephone whenever they were apart. He was sure she was having an affair. Phyllis was sure Ted was having a breakdown.

"My loving, attentive husband became a raving maniac," Phyllis recalls now. "He'd accuse me of the most horrible things, and then turn around and beg my forgiveness and dispute his own accusations. I had never seen anything like this before, so I really thought he was having some sort of breakdown. But I also felt that somehow I was to blame."

When Ted finally admitted that he was out of control, the two sought professional help. "Counseling saved our marriage," Phyllis says, "I'm convinced of it." Now, two years later, the couple has built more trust and better communication between them. Phyllis is still a busy account executive, but Ted no longer perceives her job as a threat to their marriage.

Jealousy is a dramatic emotional response to a real or imagined threat to an existing relationship. If the threat is real, such as when you find out your partner is having an affair, then jealousy is a normal reaction; but if there is no real evidence or probability of cause, then the jealousy is said to be "delusional" and, therefore, sick. One survey of marriage counselors found that jealousy was a problem for approximately one-third of all couples seeking counseling (Pines, 51).

Irrational jealousy is always indicative of deeper fears and problems, so the only hope for dealing with it is to find and attack the psychological cause. But that can be a complicated process. In Ted's case, Phyllis' job took her physically away from him, rekindling the familiar feelings of abandonment he had felt as a child. His father, a traveling salesman, had been absent for every major event in his son's life, and his mother, suspicious and insecure, had made her son share the burden of her loneliness. Ted knew Phyllis wasn't having an affair, but he accused her of it the same way his mother had repeatedly accused his father.

A certain amount of playful or feigned jealousy can be both humorous and flirtatious in a marriage. After all, everyone likes to feel prized. But the real thing, a real insidious jealousy, with or without reason, steadily erodes the foundation of trust in a relationship. It feeds on itself. Security and stability cannot prevail in an atmosphere of doubt and suspicion.

If you think you have valid reasons to be jealous, air them, not in the form of accusations, but in a calm and honest way that gives your partner a chance to explain. By the same token, if you have, even inadvertently, given your spouse reason to doubt your loyalty and affection, take the responsibility for that and be more sensitive in the future.

Little pangs of jealousy now and then are normal, if only because it's human nature to doubt that good fortune can last. But if these pangs are serious enough to be upsetting or cause emotional outbursts, then the behaviors that triggered them have to be discussed so each of you can become more aware of the other's sensitivity.

Finally, if either of you suffers from repeated bouts of delusional jealousy, get professional help fast, before it destroys you and your relationship.

Sexual Difficulties

Most couples have some sexual difficulties or concerns during their married lives; some even have major ones. The important thing for you to know at this stage is that a problem becomes a problem when it is perceived to be one, and that many potential problems can be brought under control before they get to be full-blown. You should also know that sexual difficulties are not synonymous with marital difficulties.

When you think about the complexity of the human body and the human psyche, and the delicate dance lovers must go through to experience sexual satisfaction and to reproduce themselves, it's a wonder anybody ever gets it right. Lots of couples don't, at least not all the time. Many deal with sexual dysfunction, disease, or disappointment on a regular basis, and find great relief in knowing that they aren't alone and that help is available.

Dr. Judy Seifer emphasizes a practical, commonsense point of view, however: "Most newlyweds do not need sex therapy," she says. "If anything, they need sex education, and they need to know that they are okay, that what they are experiencing is not that uncommon, and that sex will get better and better over the years." (See the Appendix for an instructional video for married couples narrated by Dr. Seifer.)

If you think you need some professional counseling or advice, you can contact the American Association of Sex Educators, Counselors and Therapists (called AASECT for short). They will provide you with a list of certified members in your area. (See the Appendix for the number.)

What follows is a brief description of the most common sexual performance anxieties, and those most likely to affect newlyweds. But before discussing them, it is important to make two things clear: first, an isolated incident does not a problem make. If you overreact, however, and make it a bigger deal than it is, you will surely turn an otherwise minor incident into a permanent problem.

Secondly, sexual desire and performance are affected by many outside influences including: stress and worry, even over the desire to get pregnant; the after-effects of surgery; physical illnesses and conditions, including hypertension, depression, and mood disorders, and all the medications used to treat them; recreational drugs, including nicotine and alcohol; and hormonal imbalances. Always investigate these causes first before leaping to the conclusion that deep psychological disturbances are at work.

See References for additional information on any performance anxiety that worries you.

Infrequency of intercourse: Don't measure yourselves against the surveys done in popular magazines. There is no such thing as a "normal" average (number of times a day, week, month, etc.) for sexual intercourse. As we've already mentioned, frequency will diminish from those hot-blooded honeymoon days but, hey, it's quality, not quantity, right? What works for you is what's normal for you, and you don't have to compare yourselves to anybody else.

Premature ejaculation: This is the most common problem of younger men, and the most common complaint of young wives, because many young men lack sexual experience and the skill and self-control that comes from sexual experience. Usually, the security of lovemaking with one partner, and the time and the privacy of one's own home, help this difficulty to subside. But, if not, there are exercises that can help. A man who is worried about premature ejaculation should see his doctor or consult a sex therapist.

Retarded ejaculation: This is the opposite of the previous difficulty; the man is able to get an erection and have intercourse, but he simply cannot ejaculate. If physiological causes have been eliminated, then this involuntary inability to ejaculate could have a psychological origin. Sex therapy is indicated if the condition is more than temporary or occasional.

Impotence: The man is unable to achieve or sustain an erection for intercourse. According to Ed Schilling, Executive Director of The Impotence Institute of America, over 30 million men suffer from chronic impotence, and many of them are under age 30. It's important to remember, though, that *every man experiences temporary impotence sometimes.* It is not usually a big deal. Impotence is termed chronic only when it persists for more than six weeks.

"Impotence is treatable," Schilling says. "Fully 80 to 85 percent of the cases are symptoms of physical, not psychological, problems, so they can be alleviated right away with the proper diagnosis." His organization offers fact sheets, educational materials, membership programs, and general information (see Appendix).

Inhibited sexual desire: This complete disinterest in sex can happen to both men and women. Its origin is often physiological, due to illness, depression, or medications (see above), but it may also be a psychological defense mechanism in response to an unpleasant sexual experience. If the condition persists, therapy is indicated.

Failure to reach orgasm: Here's the truth: the *majority* of women cannot reach a climax through intercourse alone; they must have additional clitoral stimulation. Obviously, if a woman's partner is unwilling or unknowledgeable, she will remain unfulfilled. A woman can help solve that problem by instructing her lover and showing him how to give her pleasure.

Vaginal discomfort: Failure to lubricate, unconscious muscular contractions, or other conditions that make intercourse painful are not normal. Don't suffer. See your doctor.

Sexually Transmitted Diseases (STDs)

The sad thing about sexually transmitted diseases, and the resulting infertility they can cause, is that they are preventable. Ironically, in an era of AIDS awareness and all the media emphasis on safe sex, STDs have reached epidemic proportions. Literally millions of Americans are infected already. Although women, teenagers, and minorities suffer disproportionately high percentages of sexually transmitted diseases, infection is increasing most rapidly among white, educated, sexually active men and women between the ages of 25 and 35.

"I am constantly amazed at how little concern or precaution people exercise in face of this issue," says a doctor in a Boston-area health clinic. "They don't think it can happen to them, they don't worry about it, they don't get tested, and they don't tell their regular sexual partners, often their spouses, that they too are at risk. Nobody does anything until symptoms appear, and then it may be too late."

If you or your partner has one of these conditions, you are no doubt already under a doctor's care, or should be. If either of you was sexually active before marriage, particularly with several partners, you may be at risk. The really frightening aspect of STDs is that you can be infected and not know it. What's worse is that some of these infections can be passed on to an infant should an infected woman become pregnant.

The public perception persists that "nice people" don't get social diseases, so that suspicion of infection is often accompanied by shame or guilt that inhibit seeking treatment. Put your health first. If either of you thinks you've been exposed to a sexually transmitted disease, don't wait for symptoms to appear. Call your doctor and get tested.

Here, compiled from the latest information supplied by The Alan Guttmacher Institute, a nonprofit reproductive health, research, and policy institute in New York City, are the major STDs to be concerned about:

Pelvic inflammatory disease (PID): The most common complication of STDs in women, PID is caused by a bacteria or virus that attacks the reproductive organs and can result in permanent scarring, ectopic pregnancies, and infertility. PID is often the end result of gonorrhea, chlamydia, and herpes.

Chlamydia: This bacterial infection is more common, and more dangerous, than gonorrhea, because it is difficult to detect. It occurs in both men and women. Chlamydia is treatable with certain antibiotics; untreated, it can cause PID, birth defects, infertility, and other genital diseases.

Viral infections: It is estimated that one in five Americans is infected with one of the viral STDs other than AIDS: genital herpes, human papillomavirus

(HPV, also known as genital warts), and hepatitis B. Commonly considered less serious than some of the other STDs, these viral infections nevertheless take their toll, both physically and emotionally. First of all, these conditions have no cure; they can only be monitored as physical outbreaks may come and go. Second, viral STDs are also associated with liver disease and cancer. The greatest danger is during pregnancy, especially if the condition is active in the birth canal during delivery. Infected infants can die or suffer brain damage.

These viral infections can be avoided with the use of condoms; once contracted, they can be managed with good health habits, medication, and education. During active, infective stages, sexual intercourse should be avoided. Sadly, though, the viruses may be transmitted to one's partner, even when physical symptoms are not present.

Family Planning

Your reproductive life belongs to you, and the decisions the two of you make about having children are intensely personal. Ostensibly, everyone agrees with that statement, but in reality, you're going to find that while your lovemaking may be private, the consequences of intercourse are in the public domain. "Sometimes I feel like a king's consort, under constant pressure to produce an heir," moans one newly married woman.

Invasive comments come at newlyweds from every quarter. Parents, relatives, friends, even casual acquaintances think nothing of asking you when you're going to make them grandparents, aunts, uncles, or godparents—and even less than nothing of reminding you that your biological clock is ticking away. Everybody has advice about when, how many, and how far apart, and nobody is shy about sharing it.

For most couples, such intrusions are a bother, but for couples who are having difficulty conceiving, or for those who feel forced to defend their decisions to delay or defer having children altogether, the constant questions and unwelcome opinions can become sources of anger, resentment, and pain. You'll have to steel yourselves because you can probably expect to enjoy only about a year or so of married life before you have to start telling busybodies to "MYOB."

For some couples, however, especially those with unusual health risks or those in religious, racial, or cultural intermarriages, just the opposite happens: the topic of future children is carefully avoided among the relatives and friends. In these cases, it is the news of pregnancy, even when the couple welcomes it, that presents problems because now everyone must deal with whatever intermarriage issues they were trying to ignore or postpone. For couples in these situations, the decision to have a child will never be easy and the time may never seem exactly right.

Speaking of timing, experts generally agree that a couple should wait a year or two to give their own marriage a chance to stabilize before starting a family because children will put a strain on even the best relationships. Even with planning, though, babies rarely arrive at just the right moment, and they never come equipped to raise themselves. Being a parent is the single most important job anyone can tackle, yet it is the one for which most people have the least preparation.

Making the Decision

Having a child is the most serious decision anyone can make because it's a decision that endures for a lifetime. There is simply no way to be fully knowledgeable before becoming a parent. Even if you babysat and had lots of younger siblings, minding other people's children doesn't even come close to the responsibility of having your own. And, even if you are convinced that creating new life is what love is all about, you will not be fully prepared for all the trouble and the worry that babies bundle up with their joy.

Worry and responsibility aside, however, most couples do want children one day, and with so many marrying in their late twenties and early thirties, the effort to conceive is commencing sooner rather than later in marriage. (See the section, "Putting Off Parenthood" later in this chapter.) Unfortunately, for many couples, having a baby comes down to economic choices more than anything else.

According to the U.S. Department of Agriculture, the estimated cost of raising a child to the age of 18, *without* the expense of preschool, private school, or a college education, is approximately $150,000. Add to that the loss of income, at least temporarily, if one parent decides to stay at home, or the cost of child care if not. And don't forget the big question most couples ask up front: which comes first, the baby or the house?

Although you may have discussed all this and more before the wedding, changing circumstances can make family-planning decisions some of the most difficult you'll have to make in your married life. If there are financial worries or job pressures, you'll have to determine priorities and decide what you can or cannot afford to do. If you have medical problems or health considerations, you will have to consult specialists and professionals to help you understand your options. And, if the issue of contraception or a problem pregnancy thrusts you into a moral or religious dilemma, you'll have to come to terms with that, too.

With the freedom of choice comes responsibility, even a certain amount of anxiety. In this way, perhaps, modern science has created mixed blessings for today's couples.

Contraceptive Choices

With the new methods of reversible birth control on the market, and further research being done all the time, couples today have more opportunity than ever to find effective, safe contraceptive methods that will support their family-planning decisions. Yet, for all our sophistication, Americans are notorious for the misuse of contraceptives. From The Alan Guttmacher Institute comes a staggering statistic: 10 percent of all sexually active women of childbearing age use no method of birth control at all, and more than half of all the pregnancies each year are unplanned (Harlap, Kost, and Forrest, 7).

Although no method of reversible birth control is completely foolproof or without potential side effects, both effectiveness and safety are considerably enhanced by the informed choice of an appropriate method for you and by the careful, consistent use of that method according to the manufacturer's directions. Age, health risk, duration of use, and even personal lifestyle are all factors to be considered when making your contraceptive choice, and that choice will probably have to change from time to time as your situation and family plans change.

Your gynecologist can help you understand the medical advantages and disadvantages of various methods and their suitability for you, and he or she can also keep you informed about new products on the market that might be better, more convenient, or more effective than whatever you're using. You should always reevaluate your present method with your doctor during your yearly checkup. Other considerations, such as convenience and cost, factor into the decision as well.

Some methods, particularly the barrier methods, may interfere with spontaneity, being cumbersome and easier to forget in the heat of the moment, thus becoming less reliable. Health risks scare many women away from the more effective pill or IUD. Even so, the 1992 Ortho Annual Birth Control Study, done by the Ortho Pharmaceutical Corporation, reports that the pill remains the nation's most popular contraceptive, with 28 percent, or 18.7 million women, currently using it and staying on it for an average of nearly five years.

Cost is a consideration, since most insurance plans do not reimburse for birth control and some methods, like the Norplant® implant, are expensive. Then there are the religious considerations, most notably the Catholic Church's stricture against all means of artificial birth control. Couples who choose to honor these regulations will have to rely on natural family-planning methods, some of which can be fairly reliable when properly taught and carefully monitored. Natural family planning (NFP) works best, of course, for women who have regular cycles. (By the way, NFP is often used as a tool for couples trying to conceive.) Check with a local hospital, particularly a Roman Catholic institution, for natural family planning classes being held in your area.

Ideally, contraception is a mutual decision made by both of you together. Having said that, however, it also must be said that the woman should not have to bear the sole responsibility for birth control, nor should she be the only one to take the risk or suffer the inconvenience. (Bad enough that she bears the bulk of the consequences of a method's failure.)

Contraception should never be a unilateral choice or a secret determination. It has to be discussed between you, not only because parenthood is a mutual decision, but also because satisfaction and security with the methods you use, or the determination to try to conceive, can directly affect the quality of your sex life.

A Guide to Contraception

Most women will use several different types of contraception during their reproductive lives. Here are the choices currently available to you.

The Birth Control Pill

Description: Oral contraceptives purchased in monthly packets containing synthetic hormones (estrogen and progestin) that trick the body into thinking it is already pregnant, thus eliminating ovulation. Must be taken daily.

Advantages: Convenient, effective (only a 2.5 percent failure rate), and reasonably priced. Various dosages available to minimize side effects; recent studies even indicate some health advantages to pill use. Once the pill is discontinued, most women have no trouble conceiving.

Disadvantages: Available only by prescription. Can have side effects, including weight gain and mood alteration. Not recommended for women with certain health histories, those who smoke, or those over 40.

The Intrauterine Device (IUD)

Description: The IUD is a small, T-shaped device containing either copper or the hormone progesterone. It is implanted in the uterus by a doctor and left in place for one to eight years, depending on the type of IUD used.

Advantages: Convenient and extremely effective, with a 2.5 percent failure rate. Health hazards resulting in the infamous lawsuits in the 1970s have been eliminated.

Disadvantages: Must be surgically implanted and removed; not generally recommended for younger women, those with certain health histories, or those who have not yet had children. There is a small risk of pelvic inflammatory disease, which can lead to infertility.

Contraceptive Implants

Description: The newest entry in the contraceptive market, levonorgestrel implants release synthetic progestin, which prevents ovulation, for a period of five years. As of this writing, only the Norplant System®, manufactured by Wyeth-Ayerst Laboratories, is available. It consists of six 1.3-inch capsules inserted in a fan-like pattern under the skin in the arm.

Advantages: Implants are safe (with 20 years of research behind the method), effective (with less than a 1 percent failure rate), and convenient (because protection is continuous). The low hormone dosage that is released means side effects are few, and it does not contain estrogen (which accounts for the problems many women have with the pill).

Disadvantages: A minor surgical procedure is involved in implantation; the cost, including doctor's fee, is expensive ($800 to $1,000); it is not as effective for heavier women; and it may cause minor side effects, such as weight gain and menstrual disruptions.

The Barrier Methods

The Diaphragm or Cervical Cap: These rubber domes of various sizes are used with spermicidal cream or jelly. The diaphragm is larger and is inserted to completely cover the cervical area; the cervical cap is smaller and covers only the cervix. The diaphragm is much more popular, and the cervical cap can be hard to find. Both must be sized and fitted by a doctor and obtained through a prescription. Women need instruction and practice to learn how to use them properly.

Advantages: Most women can use these methods effectively, and there are no side effects. When properly fitted and properly inserted, the failure rate is less than the reported 18 percent. Cost is extremely economical, about $20, plus the yearly doctor's checkup.

Disadvantages: Depending on the design and your dexterity, the diaphragm or the cap can be difficult and messy to insert, and difficult to remove. Furthermore, it can become dislodged during lovemaking, which obviously increases the risk of pregnancy. The barrier must remain in place six to eight hours after intercourse, and repeated intercourse necessitates that additional spermicidal cream or jelly be inserted into the vagina.

Spermicides: Readily available over the counter, spermicidal contraceptives come in various forms: in sponges (moistened to release the spermicide and inserted vaginally); vaginal suppositories (small inserts containing spermicide that dissolve in the vagina); creams, jellies, and foams (all spermicidal preparations introduced into the vagina).

Advantages: Available without prescription and relatively inexpensive, except for the sponge, which can be used only once. Easy to use and without side effects (except for minor skin irritations in some individuals who have an allergic reaction to some preparations).

Disadvantages: The products can be messy, and overall effectiveness varies, with failure rates of between 10 and 20 percent. Obviously, the effectiveness is considerably increased when spermicides are used in conjunction with a diaphragm and/or condom.

Condoms: A thin sheath of rubber or animal tissue placed over the penis to catch the sperm and prevent it from entering the vagina during intercourse. The popularity of the condom has increased dramatically due to the protection it offers against disease, so that manufacturers of the device have gotten "very creative" in their design and packaging.

Advantages: Available without a prescription and fairly inexpensive. Condoms allow men to share the responsibility for contraception.

Disadvantages: Failure rate is approximately 14 percent, mainly due to misuse. (Effectiveness is increased when used with a spermicide.) Rarely, a man experiences an allergic reaction to rubber; some men claim a loss of sensitivity and pleasure with condom use.

(Note: All the barrier methods share a common complaint: that they interrupt spontaneity. But, inventive couples can make the insertion/application of these contraceptives part of their love play.)

Natural Family Planning (NFP)

Description: Avoidance of sexual intercourse when the woman is in her fertile periods, during ovulation. Employs either monitoring the basal body temperature or vaginal mucus (or both) to determine periods of fertility. (Ovulation predictor kits are available without prescription in most pharmacies.)

Advantages: Religiously sanctioned, without health risks, and cost-free, except for a nominal fee that may be charged to take the NFP classes. Women learn more about their bodies and their natural cycles, and may be able to put this information to positive use when they are trying to conceive.

Disadvantages: Even for women with regular periods, the failure rate is high: about 24 percent. The method requires skill, intelligence, and conscientious daily monitoring to be successful, and it does mean that couples must control their sexual desire and avoid intercourse for about 10 days out of each 28-day cycle.

Sterilization

Description: Either a tubal ligation for the woman, or a vasectomy for the man. Both are surgical procedures, although the vasectomy is simpler and is performed in a doctor's office under local anesthesia. Tying off the woman's fallopian tubes is done in the hospital under general anesthesia, most easily right after the delivery of a baby. A newer procedure, the laparoscopy, is a bit simpler. These are permanent procedures; in spite of what you may have heard or read, don't count on their being reversible.

Advantages: Virtually 100 percent effective, and there are usually no side effects once performed successfully. A good choice for couples who have either completed their families, or who do not want children or should not (for medical reasons) have them.

Disadvantages: These are irreversible, fairly expensive surgical procedures.

In the Making

Description: Contraceptive research continues, and some methods available abroad may eventually gain approval for marketing in the United States. Likely newcomers in the near future include the *vaginal ring,* which releases hormones and is replaced monthly, the *male pill,* and a *contraceptive vaccine. Disposable cervical caps* and *female condoms* are also in the offing. Keep reading and stay in touch with your doctor.

Putting Off Parenthood

Conventional medical wisdom is that the average woman has about a 30 percent chance of getting pregnant in any given month, and that's if her biology is in perfect working order. Start to factor in prior medical history, lifestyle habits, age, and, well, you know the story: fertility drugs, reproductive clinics, ovulation charts, doctor specialists, and sex by the biological clock. It's every high-powered, thirty-something career woman's nightmare.

The National Center for Health Statistics reports that the number of women between the ages of 30 and 39 having their first child has more than tripled in the last ten years. Certainly, most of these women have problem-free pregnancies and normal, healthy babies, as some older, much-publicized "celebrity" moms have proven. But there are definite risks associated with pregnancy at a later age and, in order to make an informed decision about postponing parenthood, you need to know what those risks are.

The first factor, of course, is reduced fertility as you age. If you're over 30, it will probably take somewhat longer to conceive. (Age affects fertility in both sexes.) So, if your plan is to fit a pregnancy neatly into a "window of opportunity," perhaps between career moves, you'd better reconsider that plan. Mother Nature might not be as cooperative as you hope.

Once you do conceive, you should know that, being older, you have an increased risk of miscarriage, and a directly age-related risk of chromosomal abnormalities in the fetus, such as Down's Syndrome. (Tests are available to monitor fetal development and determine genetic defects, of course, but that kind of knowledge comes fraught with its own stresses and problems.) You will also be more likely to experience other complications while carrying the baby to term, and you'll have a significantly higher prospect of delivering by Cesarean Section.

Now, before you throw this book down and race to the bedroom to make a baby right away, you should also know that the case for delaying childbirth is not without its positive arguments, and that every woman who waits is not an automatic candidate for disaster. Gale A. Sloan, a registered nurse, medical writer, and author of a comprehensive book on the subject, *Postponing Parenthood,* points out that women can take active steps to "maintain their reproductive fitness" while making informed family-planning choices.

"This is a very individual decision," Sloan says, "and having children too soon, before you're financially and emotionally ready, can be just as difficult and problematic as waiting too long."

She encourages women to gather health information so they can determine what their risks are, and then to take proactive steps to protect their fertility. Such simple, commonsense precautions as quitting smoking, reducing stress, getting regular gynecological exams, and trying to lead a healthful lifestyle will all help you maximize your chances for conception later on. (See Appendix for Sloan's informative book.)

From a whispered commitment to a loving caress to the miracle of creating a new life, intimacy builds and deepens as two people become one couple. Love makes the moments happen; it's up to you to savor them, and to cherish them, together.

CHAPTER 6

Making a Home

W hile it will probably take some time to make your dream home a reality, loving attention devoted to creating a warm, welcoming environment can start the very first day you cross the threshold. As every professional decorator knows, the loveliest homes are not the most lavishly or expensively furnished; they are homes that most truly reflect the character, interests, and personalities of their occupants. Even the tiniest apartment or rental can be customized and distinguished with decorative choices that reflect who you are and what you enjoy. It is this individualization, this extension of personal style and character, that separates "making" a home from merely "decorating" one.

"Today's newlyweds are independent-minded shoppers," affirms Robert W. Nightengale, Jr., of The Home Furnishings Council. "They are sophisticated consumers who do not respond to sales pressure; rather, they expect retailers to guide them, to provide them with information, and to help them learn how to express themselves in their new home." Mr. Nightengale points out that more and more retailers are responding to those needs with in-store seminars and panel discussions designed for engaged and newlywed couples. (You might keep an eye out for such educational promotions in your area, and check the Appendix for a valuable decorating guide available from The Home Furnishings Council.)

Making a home means more than buying or renting a place to live and filling it with furniture; it means creating a haven in which you and your spouse feel equally and totally comfortable and secure, and in which your family and friends can enjoy your particular hospitality. With flair and imagination, and a little planning and common sense, your house can exude an individualized warmth and personality and become a common source of pride, pleasure, and satisfaction.

The fun, and the challenge, of setting up your first home is found in the accommodation of two styles, tastes, and habits in a single, unified, harmonious living environment. In order to successfully achieve that, you'll have to work and plan together, making compromises and considering each other's preferences and requirements while selecting all your home furnishings.

For most couples, particularly those who are "starting from scratch," this is one of the most enjoyable and exciting tasks of the newlywed period. Not only will you get to shop without guilt, for bona fide necessities, but you'll get to know each other better in the process. At last you'll be turning your fantasy of life in a love nest for two into a full-blown reality.

⚜ DO YOU SEE YOURSELF HERE? ⚜

- Are you overwhelmed by the task of setting up a home, and unsure of where to begin?
- Do you lack confidence in your own taste and sense of style?
- Do the two of you have to rectify conflicting tastes and determine a style that will work for you both?
- Are you unsure of how to integrate what you already have with what you need to purchase?
- Do you need to educate yourself about furniture styles, periods, and designs?
- Are you afraid of making costly decorating mistakes?
- Are you lacking knowledge and experience as a consumer in the home-furnishings market?
- Do you need to develop a long-range plan so that you can budget your purchases and furnish your home over time?

Yes? Read on.

More importantly, though, the way you live and the things with which you surround yourselves bespeak the values, backgrounds, and commitments the two of you share. Like everything else in your relationship, the way you make a home, and the kind of home you make, grow out of your identity as a couple and, over time, help to reinforce and project that identity. That's why it's vital that you undertake homemaking together: the life you share now belongs to you both, and you both have to have a hand in shaping it.

Designs for Living

While the professional decorator or designer may take many years to perfect a distinctive touch and a sure sense of taste and intuition, you don't have to be a professional to know what you like, what your lifestyle needs are, and what makes you comfortable. And answering those questions is where successful home decorating begins.

"Even when you're just starting out, you have to think in terms of a total home concept," says Maria Ecks-Chamberlain, Divisional Director of Home Furnishings for Burdines, the Florida retail chain. "We've thrown around the word 'lifestyle' a lot, but it's important to understand lifestyle—meaning how you're *really* going to live—so you can decorate for it. You have to ask yourselves, Will you entertain a lot? Are you outdoor people? Do you have animals, or do you or will you have children? These are crucial questions. No matter what's stylish or what's fashionable at the moment, the only trend you should follow is the one created by the way you want to live."

A Decorating How-To

With so much to choose from in the home-furnishings market today, shopping in a haphazard, nondirected way can be both costly and inconvenient. The couch that looks great in an expansive showroom can literally overwhelm a small city apartment; the plaid curtains, on sale, that you're just sure will complement the floral seat cushions in the dinette can prove ghastly when you get them home. Even paint is a different color when it dries!

To help make these decisions and avoid costly decorating mistakes, many couples rely on the advice of a professional designer, whose services are often free, by the way, at department and specialty stores where you'll be making major purchases. "Regardless of where you are and where you're starting, having a purchasing plan and using the services of a professional will take much of the guesswork out of decorating decisions and will save you money, as well," says Burdines' Ecks-Chamberlain. "People need to get rid of the intimidation they feel about working with interior designers, and to think of them as trained professional shoppers for the home."

So, you need a plan and you need a budget. Here are five steps to follow to find out where you are and where you're going. Then, use the charts, guides, and worksheets provided in this chapter to help you customize your approach and turn your house into a home.

A Five-Step Approach

Step 1: Determine your likes and dislikes. What are the favorite things each of you owns? Do they have a common style, color, or line? What kind of clothing do you wear? What rooms in parents' or friends' houses do you find particularly pleasing? Visit room displays in your favorite furniture/department stores and talk about what appeals to you, and what doesn't.

You probably did some of this when you were engaged and making your preliminary selections through the bridal gift registry. Look again at the things you chose, particularly the styles, patterns, and colors of your tabletop choices. These should give you some direction as you begin to shop for furniture, floor-coverings, wallcoverings, window treatments, and accessories.

Finally, familiarize yourselves with the wide variety of home furnishings available by going through the section "Your First Home Together" in *Modern Bride* and reading other home-furnishings catalogues and shelter magazines. Begin to collect pictures of anything and everything you like, from an entire room furnished with expensive antiques to an individual piece of furniture or an inexpensive piece of pottery. When your folder starts to bulge, you'll be able to spread all your pictures out on a table and to analyze the elements common to many of the choices you've made. This is how you start to recognize the consistency of your own style and taste.

Bring pictures of things you like with you when you shop, so that a professional in the store can interpret your preferences and educate you in the coordination of style, color, and proportion. If your tastes are truly eclectic, home furnishings specialists will also show you how disparate and dissimilar objects can, in fact, be made to work together.

Step 2: Look at what you have. Now is the time to give a serious, cold-hearted second look at whatever each of you brought to your new home from your single days. Do you really want fraternity beer mugs on the mantelpiece, or those faded twin bedspreads from the dorm in your guestroom? Chuck it, sell it, or donate it to charity, but weed out everything you are still living with that you don't like, so that you can begin to replace those things, albeit slowly and over time, with quality items that will fit your new married lifestyle.

If you've each been living on your own a while and have quality furnishings from an apartment or condo, then you will have to integrate what the two of you already own with new items and accessories that can pull everything together. Don't be too hasty in discarding good pieces, even if you don't have sufficient room for everything right away. You'll hate yourself if you sell his leather sofa for a song, only to realize a couple years from now that it would have been perfect in the den of a new house.

While you're making keep-it-chuck-it decisions, this is also the time to either pack away (at your mother's), give away (to someone who will appreciate them), or sell any wedding gifts you got that you know you'll never use. As you clean out, you'll also recommit yourselves to those things you already have that you really do like and want to continue to live with, and that's important. There ought to be a place for the things that are special to each of you, even keepsakes and mementoes that have nothing but sentimental value.

Step 3: Establish decorating priorities. "Your priorities will depend on where you are at the moment," says Ecks-Chamberlain. "If you're starting from scratch, then you'll have to get the basics: something to sleep on, sit on, and eat from. That usually means a couch, a bed, and a table with chairs. If you're older and more established, however, then your decorating needs are likely to involve integrating and filling in."

The professionals at Burdines Interiors advise couples to develop both a one-year and a five-year plan. That way, they can live with the space and let their total vision take shape bit by bit. By purchasing the most-needed elements in the most-used rooms first, then finishing those environments over time, the whole house gets done as opportunity and budget allow.

Even within this total-concept approach, however, individual purchasing priorities will still be determined by the couple's individual lifestyle. For instance, some couples may choose to tackle the areas in which they entertain (living room, dining room, kitchen, or den) first, and to leave the bedrooms, including the master bedroom and bath, until later. Other couples, those who lead a quieter lifestyle or who are perhaps a bit more romantic, might choose to do their own master bedroom suite down to the last detail before turning their attention to anything else. Only the two of you can determine the priorities that make sense for the way you live.

Use the handy checklist, provided by Burdines Interiors, at the end of this chapter to help determine priorities for each room, and to plan future purchases in a systematic, organized way.

Step 4: Shop like the professionals do. Professional decorators shop the market with a tape measure, floor plans, fabric swatches, paint chips, and a list of what a client already owns, including the manufacturer's name and a brief description of major pieces. So should you.

Begin by taking accurate measurements and drawing a floor plan of every room. (See floor plan directions and furniture templates that follow.) Then, assemble a color card for each room containing, if possible, fabric swatches of any window treatments, floorcoverings, and upholstered pieces you may already own, and paint chips and/or wallpaper samples of the shell of the room. (Directions for making color cards follow.)

You'll accumulate swatches and samples as you shop, and will be able to try them out alongside what you have on your color card. Likewise, take measurements of any furniture pieces you're considering buying, and then arrange corresponding templates on your floor plan to check for balance, scale, and traffic patterns before you buy.

Being organized and systematic in your shopping will help make furnishing and finishing your home the rewarding, enjoyable experience it ought to be. It is also the most efficient, economical way to get the decorative results you have in mind.

Step 5: Be an informed consumer. Study up before you buy, especially big-ticket items. Become familiar with the brand names in the industry and learn what constitutes quality. There may be a reason that two couches, while they appear almost identical, are priced several hundred dollars apart.

Once you have some understanding of what constitutes quality and value, resist the urge to buy because you "just love it" and stick to comparison shopping instead. If you see something you like at regular price, don't be too shy to ask the salesperson when, or if, that item might be on sale. (One advantage to working with store designers is that they will often tell you of upcoming sales.)

What Other Couples Say . . .

"I go along on home-furnishings expeditions to monitor the checkbook," says one newlywed woman, "but my husband definitely has the better eye for style, color, and proportion." Apparently, decorating a home is a joint venture for the majority of today's couples.

According to a *Modern Bride* Consumer Council Survey (Cahners, September 1992, 15–17), 79 percent of the couples interviewed decided on the decorating style of their new home together, and decisions on a furniture purchase were made jointly by 91 percent of the couples. By the way, taste selections were about evenly split among traditional styles (28 percent), contemporary styles (28 percent), and eclectic styles (27 percent).

There are some fine books on interior decorating at your library and bookstore. They can tell you as much as you want to know about the principles of interior design and the hallmarks of quality and construction. Manufacturers, retailers, and industry associations also publish some wonderful consumer-education booklets about their products and services. (See the Appendix for some of these resources.)

Professional Planning Techniques

Since stores are not in the habit of delivering furniture, floorcoverings, and draperies just so you can try them out and then return them, you have to be reasonably sure that what you purchase will work in the room you're decorating. The best way to do that is to bring the room to the store. That's what professional decorators do.

Making Floor Plans

You don't have to be a gifted artist to make serviceable floor plans, but you do have to be accurate. Get yourself a good retractable tape measure that's at least 25 feet long (generally available at hardware stores or lumber yards). It may cost you a little ($15–$20), but this is a worthwhile household investment.

Measuring your room will take some time, and it will be considerably easier if the two of you do it together. Start with the overall dimensions, called the shell, by measuring usable floor space. Then, measure and place all architectural details: windows, doors, electrical outlets, light fixtures, fireplaces, closets, counters, cabinets, and any other built-ins. All your measurements must be as close to exact as you can get them.

Once the measurements are taken, you're ready to draw the floor plan. This job is much easier, and neater, if you use 1/4-inch graph paper, available at most stationery or art supply stores. Use 1/4-inch = 1 foot scale to draw your shell and all existing details. Figure 5 shows some of the standard symbols.

A sample might look like Figure 6.

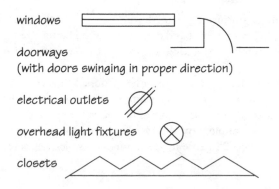

windows

doorways
(with doors swinging in proper direction)

electrical outlets

overhead light fixtures

closets

Figure 5

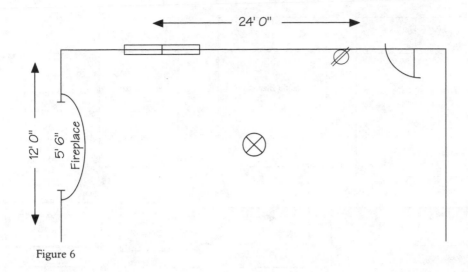

Figure 6

Furniture Templates

Once your room is drawn, you're ready to begin experimenting with various furniture pieces and placements. Photocopy the templates from Figure 7, then cut out those pieces you already own or are considering buying. (The measurements on the templates here are standard, but can easily be adapted to your needs using the 1/4-inch = 1 foot scale.)

By moving the templates around on the grid, you can see at a glance what works best where. You can consider balance, scale, and proportion, as well as the flow of traffic, and all without breaking your back moving furniture!

Making Color Cards

Color, pattern, and texture bring a room to life, and the way these elements interact makes a definite decorating statement. Style and quality in furniture and accessories are important to the personality of a room, but chances are it's the color scheme that makes the first impression.

Color affects mood, as myriad studies on the psychology of color have shown. Some tones are warm and inviting, some are stimulating and exciting, so that matching a color scheme to a room's purpose becomes an important consideration in color selection. Another consideration is proportion. Colors react to each other to appear lighter or darker, vivid or muted by comparison. Their distribution over large or small areas projects their dominance and their character in a room.

Color cards help you to match, balance, and coordinate the colors and patterns in a space. As you make choices in paint, floorcoverings, and drapery and upholstery fabrics, affix swatches and chips of those choices to the card, roughly in the same proportions as they are being used in the room itself. With the card in hand, you can evaluate new additions in light of their compatibility with everything else.

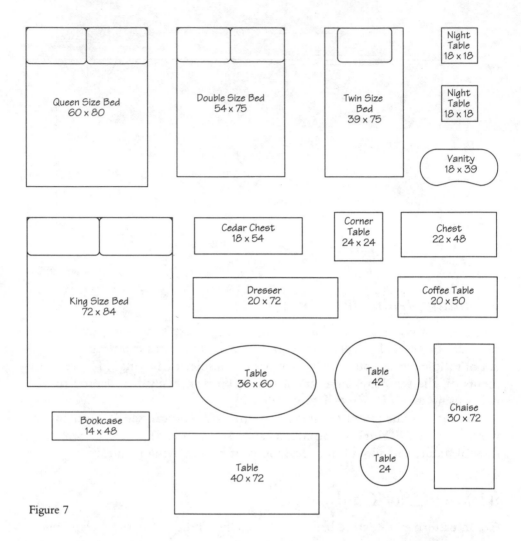

Figure 7

You can easily begin a color card of your own using the model that follows. Take a piece of plain cardboard (the backing on a legal pad would do nicely), and copy the boxes in the same sizes as Figure 8. As you shop, collect paint chips, wood finishes, fabric swatches, and carpet and wallpaper samples. As each decision is finalized, glue (or color in if samples cannot be obtained) the appropriate box in Figure 9. Just as with floor plans, an added advantage to using a color card is that it allows you to experiment with the effects of various combinations before committing yourself to the purchase.

A Quick Guide to Styles and Periods

The history of domestic styles and periods goes back to the earliest civilizations, and only major reference works on the decorative arts can do it justice. For more immediate purposes, however, here is a quick overview of the most popular styles being manufactured and reproduced today, including some of the

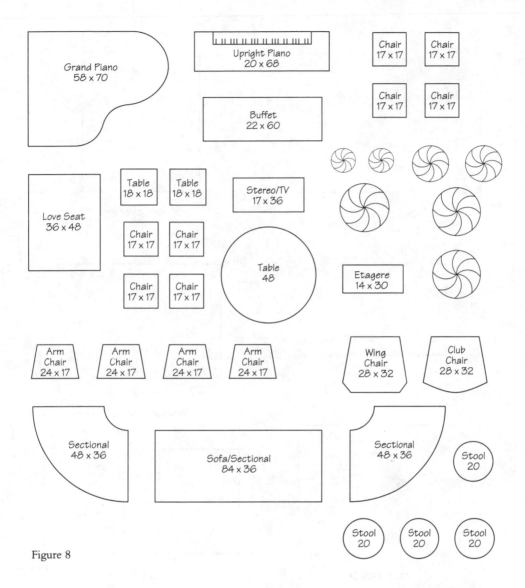

Figure 8

newest trends in American craft and regional styles. You can learn much more by attending home shows held in your area, and by studying the books on interior design in your local library and bookstore.

Traditional Styles

When we think of the classic designs of the past that have endured, we generally picture French, English, and American period pieces from the eighteenth and nineteenth centuries. The rich detailing, expert craftsmanship, and lustrous wood finishes of these highly stylized furnishings continue to be sought after and prized today, whether as period antiques or well-crafted reproductions. While traditional pieces mix well with more contemporary styles for an interesting, comfortable look, achieving an authentic period decor takes time, money, and knowledge.

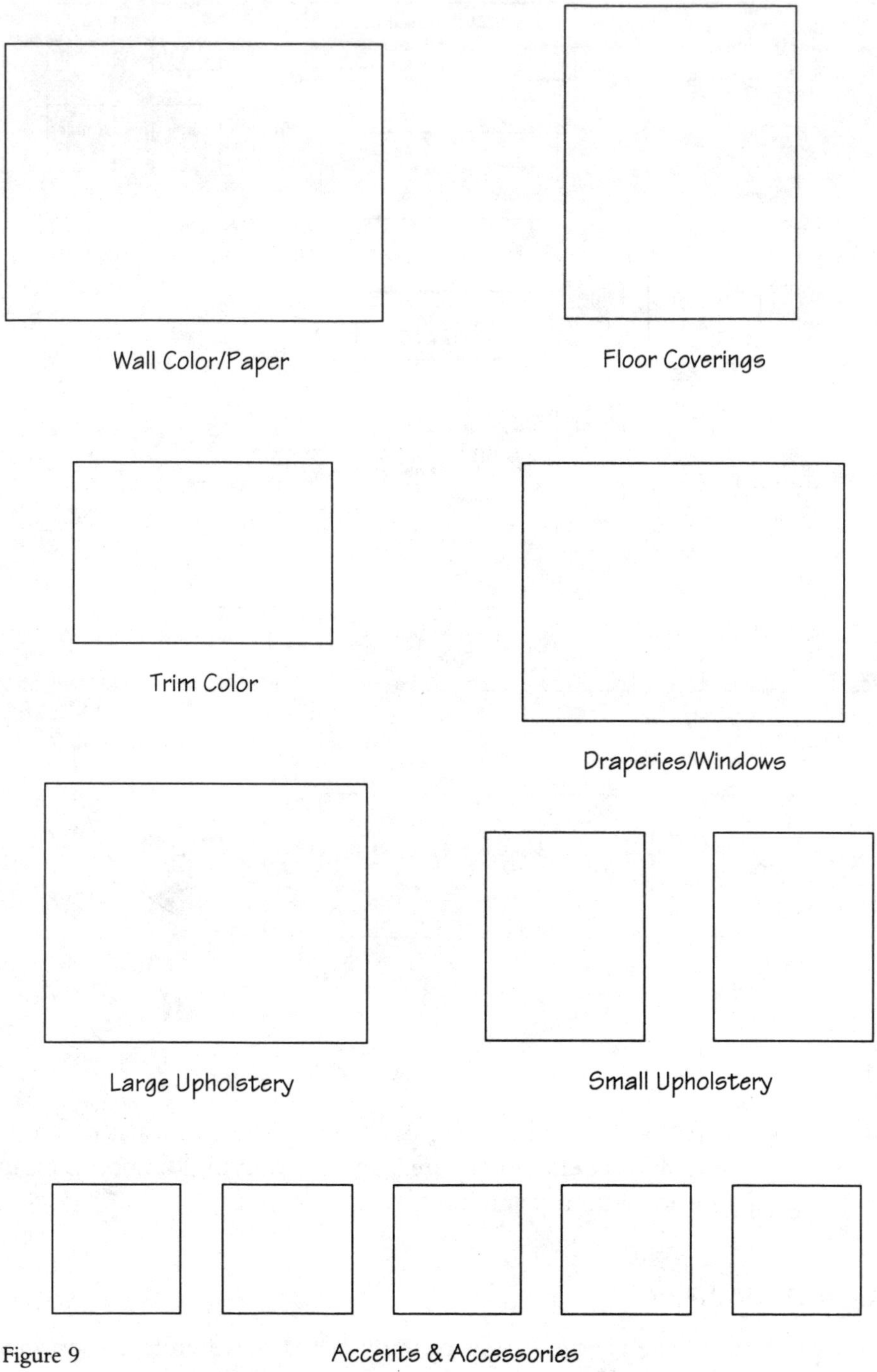

Wall Color/Paper

Floor Coverings

Trim Color

Draperies/Windows

Large Upholstery

Small Upholstery

Figure 9

Accents & Accessories

French: Includes Louis XV (1723–1774), Louis XVI (1734–1793), and Directoire/Empire (1795–1814). Lavish decoration, often gilded or lacquered, in classical motifs, such as scrolls, shells, wreaths, or crowns, characterize these stately, opulent styles. Crafted in the richest, often most exotic, woods, and upholstered in satins, silks, and brocades, traditional French styles exude formality and courtliness. The less sophisticated, less ornate French Provincial versions of the Louis styles are lighter and more adaptable to today's lifestyles.

English: Includes Queen Anne (1702–1714), Georgian (1720–1820), Chippendale (1750–1790), and Victorian (1830–1900). Generally, English furniture is symmetrical, graceful, and architecturally inspired, with the exception of the Victorian period, in which romance and nostalgia met mass production methods for some unique effects. The English designers favored mahogany, walnut, and rich wood veneers, and upholstered in softer shades of primary colors in chintz and damask. English pieces, even the antiques, seem to fit comfortably into American homes, perhaps because the British were the precursors, and the inspiration, of later American cabinetmakers and designers.

American: Includes Early American Colonial (1620–1780) and Federal (1780–1830). Basically, American designs are adaptations of English styles, but with some distinct American innovations, such as the rocking chair, the "butterfly table," the Bible box, and all kinds of chests for moving and storage. The Federal style celebrated the birth of a new republic with a richer, more formal look in dark woods with graceful lines and classic motifs. Some French influence can be seen in the work of the major American designer, Duncan Phyfe (1800–1815). American period reproductions, from Shaker chairs to New York City cabinets, are common and quite popular in the marketplace today.

Modern Styles

Some of the so-called modern styles may not seem so modern to us anymore, but the term is convenient for describing twentieth-century designs that evolved from new materials, new manufacturing methods, and new lifestyles. To the woods traditionally used for furniture crafting, for instance, were added a whole range of burls, plywoods, and veneers, as well as steel, glass, chrome, plastic, acrylic, and other synthetic materials.

Increasingly, home decorating has become a matter of creating a total environment for both living and working. As technology and electronics command a greater share of our lives and our space, the design of our homes must reflect multipurpose needs.

Art Deco (1900–1935): Shaped and directed by the iron, glass, and steel of the future, and rooted in the French Art Nouveau and "moderne" movements, the Art Deco style found its ultimate expression in the functional principles and geometric forms of Frank Lloyd Wright. Cool, graceful, and sophisticated, the Deco style has been enjoying a renaissance in popularity in late twentieth-century America.

Contemporary (1960–present): Clean, sleek, and architectural, contemporary designs are, in many ways, an extension of the modern movement and the Frank Lloyd Wright influence. Innovations by German and Scandinavian designers, who seek to integrate art with living in modular, molded, multipurpose forms, along with a migration of families back to the urban landscape, have given rise to some interesting new interpretations of what a home should look like.

High Tech (1970-present): Funky and frankly functional, this school of design is a direct result of a highly technological, space-age mentality. Clean and uncluttered, sleek and smooth, everything is unabashedly what it is, whether it's a chair, a pipe, or an exposed support beam. Materials are likely to be synthetic, and colors are usually primary and vivid against a background of white or grey.

Eclecticism (1940-present): This is a blend of styles and accessories from the past to the present, either to complement or to contrast each other, often in exciting, unexpected ways. While no one period dominates, some unifying elements (in color, form, style, or materials) are apparent. This is not just a hodge-podge, but a sophisticated mix of antique and contemporary, high tech and classic, casual and formal.

American Crafts / Ethnic Styles

With the resurgence in ethnic and regional pride, and the return to simpler values and more traditional lifestyles, the following trends are evolving and taking on new importance, and influence, in the American home-furnishings market. Even when not employed purely and completely, elements of these styles have a way of imposing themselves, in accent pieces and accessories, into a more eclectic design scheme. They are trends to watch, and to consider, in an increasingly diverse American culture.

Country: Includes Shaker, Pennsylvania Dutch, Early Colonial, and Primitive. Simple, well-constructed, almost austere furniture, except that it is sometimes decorated with handpainted or stenciled designs. Accessories include samplers and other needlework, primitive paintings and prints, braided or woven rugs, spatterware, hammered tin, and items common to country living such as milk cans, pitchers and pails, quilts, and cobbler's benches, all used in decorative ways. Also integrated into country schemes are such trendy motifs as Holstein cows, cats, pigs, and roosters.

Rustic: Includes Adirondack, Rocky Mountain, and Kentucky Log Cabin. Ponderosa pine and cedar and exposed beams characterize these styles, along with twisted-branch and twig furniture, wall-mounted antlers and hunting-lodge-type trophies, handcarved balconies, rawhide, wrought iron, washtubs, samplers, rocking chairs, and wildlife prints. Wood-burning stoves, kerosene lamps, canning jars, and Flow Blue tableware add to the "cabin" feel of these styles.

Western: Includes Santa Fe, Spanish, Mission and Hacienda, and even Pacific Northwestern. From the Far West to the California West to the Southwest, Eskimo, Native American, Mexican, and Spanish influences are evident. Characterized by adobe, tile, flagstone, and other stone surfaces, the interiors are done in earth tones, terra-cotta, animal hides, and natural fabrics.

"Santos" statues, Spanish tapestries, rough-hewn doors, Moorish arches and tiles, totem poles, masks, and other Native American tribal art, wrought iron, woven rugs, clay pots, and ceramics give an individualistic ethnic/regional twist to earthy, simple environments.

Tropical/Colonial: Includes Nantucket, Key West, Caribbean Colonial, and Miami Deco. West Indian influences prevail. Characterized by the pineapple motif, wicker, rattan, four-poster beds with mosquito netting, and cane planter's chairs. Colors are muted, cool and tropical, and formal furniture is in mahogany, in the English style. Overhead fans, tile floors, breezy fabrics, wrap-around porches, and tropical plants are just some of the accoutrements of these styles.

Miami Deco: Takes its inspiration from the Art Deco style of the thirties, when wealthy, stylish Northeasterners fled south to Miami Beach for the winter months. That style was adapted and interpreted with a tropical flavor to include pastel colors (most notably turquoise, mauve, grey, and white), glass bricks, overhead fans, marble and tile, sheer fabrics, exotic flowers and plants, and the more typical, geometric furniture.

Oriental: Includes Japanese, Chinese, and Pacific Rim influences. Simple furnishings employing clean lines and/or elegant detail in polished wood, lacquer, and inlaid surfaces, achieving uncluttered interiors. Bamboo, paper, mats, screens, sliding doors, private gardens, and Oriental art and sculpture give a serene, meditative quality to most Orientally inspired homes.

Decorating Tips

Only experience, and sometimes formal study, can teach you everything you need to know to tackle the many jobs of putting a home together, but whether you're renovating, decorating, or both, these tips might be helpful to remember as you face your own challenges.

- Every room must have a major focus, called a focal point, to which the eye is drawn and around which everything else is arranged. Usually, the focal point is an architectural feature, such as a fireplace or a large window with a great view, but a focal point can be created where one does not naturally exist. A wall grouping of artwork or photographs, a dramatic drapery treatment on otherwise unremarkable windows, a floor-to-ceiling bookcase or wall unit, or a spectacular piece of furniture could become focal points for any room.

- Repeating patterns, lines, or colors in upholstery fabrics, wallpaper borders, floorcoverings, throw pillows, picture mattings, etc., creates rhythm and unity in a room. Repetition of a theme is a great way to tie dissimilar elements together.

- Build a color scheme from the combination found in a single printed fabric, a piece of pottery, or a work of art. That way, you can be sure the overall color scheme will work, but can adjust the proportions of color to suit your own taste and needs.

- Play with proportion and distribution of color. The most interesting rooms employ at least three colors: one, called primary, dominating the largest surfaces; another playing a secondary role; and a third used as an accent. (Neutrals, grey, black, beige, and white, generally don't count.) You can carry the same scheme throughout your house, but can avoid monotony by changing the roles of each color from room to room, that is, letting an accent color in one room become the dominant color in another. Such color coordination throughout your home assures adaptability and versatility to new spaces when you move to a new home.

- Use color to trick the eye. A bright, dark, or patterned ceiling, for instance, appears lower than a light one. If you want a high-ceiling look, paint the walls a much darker color than the ceiling; if you want walls and ceiling to appear to be an exact match, you have to use a slightly lighter shade of the wall color on the ceiling. For architectural definition, paint doors, trim, and moldings a different color from the walls.

- Use texture to increase visual and tactile appeal, as well as to conceal and camouflage. Smooth or shiny surfaces reflect light and, therefore, seem cool and glamorous. They also disclose every bump and bulge. If your walls are less than perfect, use flat finish paint or wallcovering, or consider surface paint that is textured with sponges, brooms, or brushes. Flat weave and nubby textures in fabrics feel warmer and invite snuggling.

- Horizontal lines (in long, low furniture, chair rails, printed fabrics or wallcoverings) make rooms look wider; vertical lines (arches, accented doorways, floor lamps, tall furniture, bookcases, or vertical striped patterns) make a room look taller. As you pick patterns and arrange furniture, be aware of the invisible line your eye will follow as you enter the fully decorated room. Is it pleasing?

- Use room dividers, folding screens, or tall bookcases to divide space or create areas, such as an entrance hall or office space, where none exists. Portable dividers such as these make particular sense for renters, because you can take them with you. Area rugs can also be used to define space, and they, too, make more sense than installed carpeting for those who rent.

Stretching the Budget

"My advice about home decorating is walk softly and carry a big credit card," jokes Glenda, who says she's constantly postponing one purchase because another is unexpectedly high. "No matter how much you budget," she cautions, "it won't be enough. At this rate, I doubt if our house will even be done before the kids go off to college—and we don't even have the kids yet!"

Another *Modern Bride* Consumer Council study among newlyweds (Cahners, July 1993, 9) shows that couples plan to spend an average of $6,000 decorating their homes in the first year of marriage. In truth, that isn't as much as it sounds like when you consider that fancy draperies for a window wall could run up to that figure. But then again, maybe Glenda is right: no matter how much money you have to spend, it won't seem nearly enough when you discover the fabulous choices and magnificent home products available today.

The best and most obvious way to stretch your home-furnishings dollars is to avoid costly mistakes by planning carefully, getting expert advice, educating yourself in the marketplace, resisting impulse buying, and doing some comparison shopping. Beyond the tactics we've already discussed, however, here are a few other money-saving ideas.

- Continue to use your bridal gift registry. Not only is the bridal gift registrar in most stores a knowledgeable resource for decorating advice, but the gift registry itself can be enlarged, expanded, and used over several years of your early married life. Encourage your family and friends to continue to make their gift purchases for you through the registry for birthdays, anniversaries, and other special occasions. That way, they'll be sure their gifts fit into your overall decorating scheme.

- Paint is the least expensive way to get dramatic decorating results. You can bring contrast to a ho-hum room by painting one wall, or that wall and the ceiling, a different color. You can add architectural detail with borders, stripes, or geometric designs, or even paint a rug on the floor! If you're just a little bit arty-crafty, you might even try your hand at some of the great new stenciling, marbling, or free-form techniques being demonstrated at home shows around the country.

- If you have any proficiency in the domestic arts, use them. If you can sew, then order coordinated fabric with your wallpaper and make your own tablecloths, pillow shams, etc. If you can make draperies or slipcovers, you can save yourself a fortune; even if you don't sew well, you can still make simple curtains or cover throw pillows. Fabric stores often give workshops in sewing for the home (usually at night because everybody works during the day), and all the major pattern companies have tons of fantastic home-decorating projects in the back of their pattern books. Check them out.

- Likewise, if you're into crafts or woodwork, or have always wanted to be, you can get some very stylish results for little cash outlay if you can refinish furniture, build your own bookcases, hand-stencil window shades, strip and refinish floors, etc. This just might be the time to consider a new hobby.

- Next to paint, fabrics are the most economical, effective budget stretchers, and bedsheets are the most economical fabric buys. Use them for curtains, pillows, slipcovers, vanity skirts, occasional table covers (and dinner tablecloths and napkins, as discussed in Chapter 3).

- Do the "grunt work" yourselves. Even if you're not especially talented in the home arts, you can invest sweat and elbow grease in those basic, back-breaking jobs that most homes demand: painting, stripping, staining, refinishing, wallpapering, repairing, insulating, etc. Think of it this way: whatever you can do competently for yourselves will leave you that much more money to spend on the fine furnishings and highly skilled labors you cannot duplicate.

- If you have a patio and spend lots of time outside, think about investing in stylish, good-quality outdoor furniture first. In the warm-weather months, you'll probably do most of your entertaining outside anyway, and much of today's outdoor designs adapt wonderfully well to indoors in the cooler seasons. You can also find inexpensive pieces in wicker, straw, and molded plastic that will suffice for now and become nice porch/patio pieces later on.

Accessorize!

Speaking of budget stretchers, nothing will give you more mileage for the dollar than carefully chosen, well-designed, tasteful accessories. And many of the most popular accents, like potted plants and family photographs, cost next to nothing when compared to the overall character and distinction they bring to any decor.

"Our mission is to find well-designed items from all over the world that will complement and pull styles together," says Jim Prucha, Vice President of Merchandising/Accessories for Pier I Imports. "Furniture accessories and small lifestyle pieces are economical, versatile investments, especially in a new home because, as the marriage matures, accents in one room—say wicker chairs or occasional tables—can be moved elsewhere for new functions." Prucha notes that earth tones, neutral fabrics, and natural products are particularly popular today, no doubt reflecting the concern with earth and ecology, but that quality and craftsmanship never go out of style, regardless of current trends.

From ethnic crafts to dried flowers to wall hangings to rugs, it's the accessories, and the way you use them, that make a statement and assert your own personal style. And, accessories don't have to be expensive, or exotic, or even particularly unusual to do that successfully. Personal collections, family mementoes, handcrafts, local arts and crafts picked up on vacation—any of these could make distinctive additions to your home and help tie other elements together. In fact, it really is the way you accessorize, more than anything else, that gives your home the individual character and style that makes it you.

With the return today to cultural roots and tradition, and the resurgence of pride in ethnic and regional heritage, why not start thinking about the kinds of characteristic home accessories the two of you could accumulate that would reflect who you are and inform the way you live? "You don't have to make a major financial investment in order to have artwork in your home," Prucha advises. "You just have to choose carefully, and remember to keep things simple. That way, the accessories you choose will enjoy a place of prominence and make a statement."

Checklist from Burdines Interiors
"All the Comforts of Home"

Use this checklist to assess what you already own and to plan for what you need. By doing some comparative shopping, you can begin to set a realistic home-decorating budget and an estimated time frame for future purchases.

Kitchen   Price

CASUAL DINNERWARE
1-20-pc. dinnerware set .... ☐ _____
1-5-pc. completer set .... ☐ _____
1-20-pc. flatware set .... ☐ _____
1-Hostess set................................. ☐ _____
1-6-pc. glass set .... ☐ _____

COOKWARE
1-Cookware set .... ☐ _____
1-Teakettle .... ☐ _____
1-Microwave set.............................. ☐ _____
1-Kitchen tools set .... ☐ _____
1-Colander .... ☐ _____
1-Mixing bowl set .... ☐ _____
1-Glass bakeware set .... ☐ _____

ELECTRONICS
1-2 or 3 slice toaster .... ☐ _____
1-Toaster/convection oven .... ☐ _____
1-Electric can opener .... ☐ _____
1-Steam iron .... ☐ _____
1-Ironing board .... ☐ _____
1-Coffee/Espresso maker................ ☐ _____
1-Blender/Food Processor .... ☐ _____
1-Mixer... ☐ _____
1-Juice extractor .... ☐ _____
1-Sandwich maker .... ☐ _____
1-Bread maker .... ☐ _____
1-Vacuum cleaner .... ☐ _____
1-White 10" TV................................ ☐ _____
1-Cordless phone .... ☐ _____
1-Paddle fan .... ☐ _____

TABLE/KITCHEN LINENS
1-Informal tablecloth....................... ☐ _____
1-Formal tablecloth .... ☐ _____
4-Place mats.................................. ☐ _____
8-Napkins .... ☐ _____
4-Dish towels .... ☐ _____
2-Pot holders .... ☐ _____
2-Oven mitts .... ☐ _____

HOLLOWARE
1-Salad bowl/tools .... ☐ _____
1-Serving tray................................. ☐ _____
1-Candlestick set .... ☐ _____
1-Pitcher .... ☐ _____
1-Salt & pepper set .... ☐ _____

CUTLERY   Price
1-Cutlery set .... ☐ _____
4-Steak knives .... ☐ _____

MISCELLANEOUS
1-Cook book.................................. ☐ _____
1-Wooden dish rack........................ ☐ _____
1-Canister set .... ☐ _____
1-Kitchen gadgets.......................... ☐ _____

Family room/guest room
1-Sleep sofa.................................. ☐ _____
1-Sheets/cases set .... ☐ _____
1-Standard blanket .... ☐ _____
2-Pillows .... ☐ _____
1-Mattress pad............................... ☐ _____
2-Lamps .... ☐ _____
2-End tables.................................. ☐ _____
1-Wall unit/desk .... ☐ _____
1-TV/VCR/stereo............................ ☐ _____
1-Basic phone............................... ☐ _____
1-Paddle fan .... ☐ _____

Guest bath
2-Bath towels................................ ☐ _____
2-Hand towels................................ ☐ _____
4-Washcloths .... ☐ _____
4-Fingertip towels........................... ☐ _____
1-Tub mat .... ☐ _____
1-Shower curtain/liner .... ☐ _____
1-Rug.. ☐ _____
1-Wastebasket............................... ☐ _____
1-Tissue holder .... ☐ _____
1-Soap dish .... ☐ _____

Dining room
1-Dining table................................ ☐ _____
6-chairs.. ☐ _____
1-Buffet.. ☐ _____
1-Side board .... ☐ _____
1-Overhead lighting .... ☐ _____
1-Paddle fan .... ☐ _____

Living room
1-Sofa.. ☐ _____
2-Chairs .... ☐ _____
2-End tables.................................. ☐ _____
1-Cocktail table .... ☐ _____
2-Table lamps .... ☐ _____

	Price		Price
1-Entertainment center	☐ _____	1-Blanket	☐ _____
1-Area rug	☐ _____	1-Comforter/duvet	☐ _____
1-Portable phone	☐ _____	1-Bedspread	☐ _____
1-Paddle fan	☐ _____	1-Dust ruffle	☐ _____
		2-Pillows	☐ _____

Kids' bedroom

		1-Mattress pad	☐ _____
2-Twin beds/bunk beds	☐ _____	1-Portable phone	☐ _____
1-Dresser	☐ _____	1-Paddle fan	☐ _____
1-Desk	☐ _____		

Master bathroom

1-Bookcase/TV/VCR	☐ _____	4-Bath towels	☐ _____
2-Pillows	☐ _____	4-Hand towels	☐ _____
2-Sheet sets	☐ _____	8-Washcloths	☐ _____
2-Comforters	☐ _____	2-Tubmats	☐ _____
2-Mattresses	☐ _____	1-Shower curtain	☐ _____

Master bedroom

		1-Shower curtain liner	☐ _____
1-Bed	☐ _____	1-Rug	☐ _____
1-Mattress/box spring	☐ _____	1-Wastebasket	☐ _____
1-Chest	☐ _____	1-Tissue holder	☐ _____
1-Dresser & Mirror	☐ _____	1-Soap dish	☐ _____
1-Night stand & table	☐ _____	1-Scale	☐ _____
1-Chair	☐ _____	1-Hamper	☐ _____
2-Lamps	☐ _____	2-Beach towels	☐ _____
1-Clock radio	☐ _____		

Balcony & patio

1-TV/VCR	☐ _____	1-Folding chair & lounge	☐ _____
2-Sheet sets	☐ _____	1-Small table & pool accessories	☐ _____
2-Pillowcase sets	☐ _____		

Reprinted with permission.

CHAPTER 7

Pursuing Your Careers

L et's say that you have an advanced degree, that you studied hard and worked hard to be where you are today, and that you never wanted to do anything other than what you are doing professionally right now.

Doesn't matter; marriage will change the way you see your profession.

Let's try another scenario: let's say that you have a job you hate with a boss you loathe, a mindless position that pays good money, but doesn't challenge anything other than your patience.

Doesn't matter; marriage will change the way you view that situation, too.

It's called perspective. When there are two of you instead of just one, your perspective about everything else in your life, including and maybe most especially your work, changes to accommodate the new priorities you have set together. Suddenly, the decision to leave a job, or to take a promotion, or relocate, or go back to school will affect someone besides yourself, and so the decision must be made with that someone and the consequences on your relationship kept in mind.

Sometimes, the decisions are easier to make with the loving support of a spouse, and with the fall-back position of his or her income. But, sometimes, the needs of your marriage conflict with your individual career aspirations, and then the decisions are much harder to make, and maybe harder still to live with.

Work is a fact of life—for most of us, a fact of a lifetime. We may not like those economic realities, but we have to live with them. According to the Bureau of Labor Statistics, 72 percent of all married women between the ages of 25 and 44 work, and according to the latest *Modern Bride* surveys, 92 percent of all newlywed women are employed, with another 3 percent in school full-time preparing for work. And women, more than men, are concerned about the rigors of juggling work life and home life.

No doubt some of these women are devoted to careers they love, some of them labor in jobs they hate, and many feel a certain ambivalence toward work altogether—just as their husbands do. Nevertheless, today, both spouses are likely to be employed because they have to be, because it simply takes two incomes to make it, much less to get ahead. And that means each spouse has to deal not only with the job pressures of his or her own position, but also with the stresses, pressures, and demands work places on the partner.

The role of work in both your lives, and the compromises and trade-offs that have to be made because of your occupations, is an ongoing and extremely

---

ꙮ **DO YOU SEE YOURSELF HERE?** ꙮ

- Have you felt the pressure of conflicting demands between your job and your marriage?
- Does the nature of your profession(s) create inordinate demands on your time and attention?
- Does there seem to be some career competition between you?
- Do you have trouble leaving work at work and being loving and supportive at home?
- Is either of you at a juncture where it's time to rethink your career/educational goals and reassess where you're going?
- Have you been surprised by a growing ambivalence toward your career since your marriage?
- Has geographic relocation, the threat of layoff, company reorganization, or other job instabilities brought added stress to your marital relationship?
- Is one of you struggling with the difficulties of being unemployed?
- Do you as a couple live with some unusual pressures because of an extremely stressful, high-risk job?

Yes? Read on.

---

influential component of your marital partnership. Do you live to work, or work to live? What's more important, your marriage or your job? Whose job comes first? Whose career aspirations have to be sacrificed in a pinch?

These are tough questions that each of you will ultimately have to answer for yourself, but your life together will be easier if you can arrive at some compatible answers. It's important to remember, though, that the connection between work and marriage goes both ways: that is, although job stress may add pressures to your marital relationship, the security of a good marriage and an understanding partner can also make a stressful work life much easier to bear.

Life in the Fast Lane

Everybody's busy, incredibly busy. All this busyness has created a generation of what one New York psychologist has dubbed "career kamikazes" bent on successful self-destruction. Living to work or working to live is a crucial dilemma, especially in an achievement-oriented society like ours. Without a doubt, work is important, but is it everything? And, if it is, do we then have the right to ask others to play only secondary roles in our lives?

She's an environmental lawyer, he's in charge of special events for a well-known nonprofit organization. On a typical day, she's up and out by 7:30 A.M., and not back home until 8 or 9 in the evening. He leaves at little later, around 9 every morning, and arrives back home somewhere between 9 and 10 P.M. "I'm sorry it's been so hard to get together," she apologizes, when the three of us finally manage to talk at 11 o'clock at night. "But, you know, this is just the way we live."

This couple is Lori and Tim, but it could be any of the thousands of other young married couples who bring high energy and high expectations to their hopes for the future. Their resumes may differ, their schedules may vary, and the difficulties they face might be peculiar to them, but all of today's couples seem driven by the same desire: to be at least as well off as their parents were, with marriages that are even better. It's the updated version of the American Dream, and today's couples are willing to work, twice as hard if they have to, to achieve it.

"This is the way our lives are," Tim says, "and this is the way our lives are going to be, and that's okay. When I think of our parents, whew . . . both of us come out of very comfortable, high-achieving backgrounds . . . well, we'll have to work harder maybe to match that. But we've been given the tools, the drive, and the education, and so this is life for our generation. And it's a good life, and we're not complaining." He pauses for a minute and then laughs. "Well, maybe we complain a little sometimes."

"Yeah, right," Lori scoffs. "He complains because he has to kill an hour or two playing racketball a couple nights a week before I get home. Isn't that too bad. . . ."

Actually, Lori and Tim are pretty upbeat about their hectic lives and don't seem to have many complaints. In fact, just the opposite: they seem grateful. Each talks with enthusiasm about the personal satisfactions and fulfillment their respective careers offer; they freely admit that they are well compensated financially for the long hours they put in; and they appreciate the advantages those paychecks afford in terms of a nicely furnished apartment in a good area, weekend trips and luxury vacations, regular dinners out, and other leisure activities.

"You don't resent working hard and living at such a pace if you feel you're accomplishing something and getting somewhere, both professionally and personally," Tim says. "And we feel we are. We're doers, and this is the lifestyle we both want and that we're both accustomed to."

The Trade-Offs

Even so, life in the fast lane exacts a price, and Lori and Tim know it. Their one complaint, when they allow themselves the luxury of complaining, is the heavy demand their lifestyle exacts on their time and energy. Both regret that they have so little time together during the week, perhaps only two or three hours a day, and both admit that those hours are usually at night when it's not easy to be pleasant and attentive, much less romantic, after a long day.

"One of the biggest adjustments of married life for me has been that I want the limited time I have with Tim to be close and special, but I also need time to myself to unwind and get the uglies out. I never have that," says Lori. "When you're single, even when you're engaged, you always have the option of going home, going to bed, not seeing or talking to anybody if you don't want to. But when you're married, that person is there and you have some responsibility to him, to his needs, no matter how you feel or what kind of day you've had."

It's difficult to muster interest and attention when you're tired, but particularly difficult when you've had an unusually trying day. On such days, Lori confesses that her mind will wander when she and Tim talk, or that she'll fail to be sympathetic about some issue at work that he thinks is important, especially if she has just dealt with what she considers to be a really pivotal environmental issue. "The question of whose needs are greater at any given moment, and what emotional reserves the other can draw on to meet those needs, is sort of ongoing," she says.

Tim jumps in: "When you live like we do, I think you come to appreciate each other's time and effort more, the things you do for each other, the ways you put yourselves out, because you know you each have so little time and energy to spare. And you become *very* protective of your weekends. You count on the weekends to get back in touch."

When Lori and Tim look down the road five years or so, they see life as being pretty much the same way as it is now. "Oh, we might have a few more financial obligations then, especially if we've bought a home or started a family," says Tim.

"And we might have different jobs, although in the same careers," adds Lori, "and hopefully I won't still be commuting to work." But they figure it's "always going to be like this" because they're basically busy, happy people who enjoy many interests and who want to make important contributions with their lives.

"One thing for certain about the lifestyle we've chosen," Tim says. "We can't say we'll ever be bored."

The Tyranny of Time

Who would have thought, back in the idyllic days of childhood when it seemed as if we had all the time in the world, that we would all grow up to be White Rabbits forever chasing the clock? Yet, that is exactly what has happened. Time, and the stress that time pressures create, have become the universal lament of our age.

Time management experts are quick to point out that each of us, no matter who we are or what we do, has the same, finite 24-hour-a-day allotment of time. Why, then, are some people able to accomplish so much more than others with their allotment? And, more importantly, how do couples who feel acutely pressured by the demands of career, spouse, family, and personal needs manage to beat the clock without being beat all the time?

Emilio and Mary Anne are another typical professional couple. Emilio owns his own business, a successful fast-food franchise, and is soon to open another. Mary Anne is an intensive-care nurse specialist, recently promoted to head of ICU at a local hospital. They have been married two years, own a small home, and have lots of supportive, though sometimes demanding, friends and relatives in the area. Time, already in short supply before their marriage, has become an even more precious commodity after their marriage.

"Somehow, Emilio and I thought getting married would give us more time together, not less," says Mary Anne. "But it didn't work out that way. Marriage seemed to create new obligations, new needs and demands that neither of us had faced before when we had only our single selves to worry about. So we got on this treadmill right after the honeymoon, and didn't realize it until we had to postpone the celebration of our first anniversary three times!"

There is a tendency, once you're married and don't have to schedule your dates anymore, to overlook the need for scheduling altogether, even though the demands of your professional, and family and social, lives probably haven't diminished at all. The fact that the two of you are living together creates the illusion that you're seeing more of each other when, in fact, all you really may be doing is sleeping in the same bed. The more active the two of you are, and the more established your individual professional lives, the more you'll have to plan time for each other.

The difficulty of trying to arrange an anniversary date with each other brought Emilio and Mary Anne to this realization in a hurry. "It was scary to admit that, even as newlyweds, we had already put the relationship on hold while we tended to everything and everyone else first," says Mary Anne. "We didn't want to be a couple leading parallel lives, yet we each felt tremendous time pressures in meeting our individual work and family responsibilities. Something had to give, and we knew it meant rearranging our priorities."

It's not always easy to say "no" to others, to recognize what really matters, or to avoid the "robbing Peter to pay Paul" approach to time management. Only by analyzing the demands placed on you and by setting conscious priorities of your own can time really be controlled and the stress of busy lives appreciably reduced. Matters that shout urgency are not necessarily urgent, or even important.

Mary Anne and Emilio began organizing their time by putting each other at the top of their priority list. Luckily, Mary Anne's recent promotion meant that she now had a regular work schedule. Emilio agreed to shift more job responsibility to his new associate manager so he could be home when Mary Anne was. True, many of those evenings were spent doing routine chores around the house, but at least they were spent together. And, the couple set Friday nights aside for a special "date" each week.

Work and family obligations came next on the couple's priority list. Since both have demanding jobs and demanding families, they realized that careful attention had to be paid to scheduling. They posted an oversized calendar in their kitchen so they would be aware of each other's obligations, and then asked family and friends to give them a little more advance notice of special events and get-togethers so they could be sure to arrange the time to participate.

"Just talking about our schedules and discussing our personal problems with time made us both feel better," says Emilio. "It made each of us think about how we could eliminate unnecessary busywork and how we might perform necessary tasks more efficiently."

It may not be possible to literally *make* more time, but it is possible to learn to use what you have more efficiently.

Learning to Live a Little

"Planning ahead is fine, provided you don't then become driven by the schedule and create even more stress for yourself," says Mary Anne. "At some point, you have to sit down and ask yourselves what you're hurrying toward."

For Emilio and Mary Anne, the question prompted an in-depth discussion of their long-range goals and an objective reassessment of their short-term obligations. In the process, they were able to rediscover their basic values and to pat themselves on the back for some accomplishments, both personal and professional, so far.

"We realized that we often assumed obligations for friends and family members that didn't really belong to us, and that we still had difficulty saying no to every request. Once we took the long view and gave ourselves a little credit for where we are and what we've done, we were able to gain a broader perspective and to cultivate a more relaxed attitude about time," explains Emilio. "And you know what? Miracle of miracles, there's finally some free space on that calendar!"

One of the paradoxes about time is that those who have a friendly attitude toward it seem to have more of it, and those who fear it seem to have less. Psychologists tell us that most time pressures are self-imposed, more a matter of attitude than allotment. Our other busy couple, Lori and Tim, for instance, while certainly aware of the value of time and the absence of enough of it in their lives, don't seem as threatened and pressured by time constraints as Emilio and Mary Anne were.

Tim and Lori are willing to accept the hectic lifestyle their multiple goals and obligations create, and even thrive in it. They live largely one day at a time, try not to worry unduly about tomorrow, and make it a point to appreciate each other and the moments they have together. Weekends and vacations are used to rejuvenate and to reconnect with each other, family, and friends.

Emilio and Mary Anne could discover more free time on their calendar only when they quit chasing the future, started paying attention to the present, and let go of some of the guilt they had always associated with having time for themselves. More relaxed attitudes resulted because less energy was spent in worrying about what they *had* to do or *should* be doing.

Let's face it: neither of these couples, no matter how they adjust their attitudes, will find enough hours every day to do everything they would like to do. That's just part of the compulsion of being the high-energy, high-achieving people they are. But they can, if they try, carve out time here and there for puttering in the garden or reading a book or strolling hand-in-hand in the park. And so can you.

Conflicting Loyalties

"I preferred not to marry another physician," admits Simon. "In fact, when Denise and I met during training, I was reluctant to start dating her, even though we were obviously attracted to each other, because I just didn't want to get involved with someone in medicine."

But he did get involved. The attributes and attitudes that drew them to the same profession drew them to each other as well. Simon and Denise, both pediatricians, dated for two years during their residencies and have now been married two years. They feel that it's taken them longer to adjust to marriage, to set up a home, and to do the "normal" things other newlywed couples do because of the physical and emotional demands of their profession.

"To begin with, this is really the first year since we've known each other that we sort of have regular hours—or at least I do," Denise says. "I'm now in private practice, so that's a little saner, and I see mostly well children, which is much less stressful than the seriously sick and dying children you work with routinely in a hospital setting."

Simon, however, works in a clinic during the day and an emergency room at night, so he still comes home with a considerable amount of tension. "We have rules," he explains. "The person with the most frustrating day, usually me, gets to vent first, but there's a time limit. And then we set another time limit overall for how long we can talk about medicine. And then we force ourselves to go on to something else. If you don't consciously do that when you're both in the same occupation, then there's no escape for either of you. Yes, you're committed and you care about your patients, and you need to talk about that, but you have to have a break from it."

Medicine is one of those all-encompassing occupations that demand total dedication and create a total identity. There are others, too, mostly service professions, that elicit such complete mental and emotional involvement while on the job that it's virtually impossible to turn off that intensity when the day is done. While the level of commitment and performance is admirable, the danger is that life for professionals in such fields can easily become one-dimensional. Once that happens, others—spouses and children—find themselves relegated to secondary roles.

"Being in identical fields gives us each a unique understanding of what the other is going through at any time," Denise says, "and so we can help each other unwind in ways that maybe couples who don't share the same profession can't."

"I don't know," Simon teases. "I still think I should have married a high-powered lawyer, if for no other reason than conversational variety."

Temporarily Sidetracked

Claudia and Jim, in their thirties and married three years, both have MBAs and both are investment bankers—at least they both were until Claudia had the baby. For the last five months, she's been home. Now she's at the crossroads: will she return to work next month when her six-month extended maternity leave is up?

"I can't tell you how ambivalent I am about this," Claudia confesses. "On the one hand, we really need my income, I miss a lot of my clients and friends at the office, and Jim and I seem to be on different wavelengths now that I'm at

Talking Tough about Your Work Life

If stress at work creates stress at home, nothing will change unless you're honest about your situation and your own attitudes. Here are some tough questions to ask yourselves, individually, so you can assess the risks and tackle the challenges your career(s) poses to your marital relationship.

1. Are you in a high-stress, nontraditional or non-9-to-5 occupation: medical professions, law enforcement, firefighter or emergency services, teacher, lawyer/litigator, competitive brokerage, etc.?
2. Has your work been a primary source of personal satisfaction, self-identity, and self-esteem?
3. Do you feel your career is "more important," in terms of position, prestige, potential, or income, than your spouse's?
4. Is yours a highly competitive field, so that you're under constant pressure to be faster, better, smarter to get ahead?
5. Do you work late often, or do you routinely bring work home in the evenings and on weekends?
6. Are you expected to devote a significant amount of your leisure time to entertaining clients or socializing with colleagues?
7. Are you unable to take all of your vacation, two weeks or more, at one time each year if you wanted to?
8. Are any of the following necessary for your work: a beeper/pager, a car phone, a home fax machine, a home computer/modem, a separate business telephone in your home?
9. Are you self-employed?
10. Are your present work-life patterns likely to continue throughout your career and your married life?

There is no score for this inventory because you can't flunk; you can only fail to take the number of yes answers you have seriously. The more yesses, the more likely you are to be, or to become, a workaholic, and the more your work is apt to jeopardize, or at least interfere with, your personal life.

home with the baby and the dog all day. He doesn't talk to me about the deals he's doing the way he used to and, you know what's worse, I don't even ask."

She frowns, then continues. "On the other hand, I really don't feel much like an investment banker myself anymore, and I'm just not sure pushing paper and making deals is all that important in the big scheme of things. I worry about my son growing up without me, particularly in these early years, and the child care hassles make me tired already, and I haven't even started them yet. But then I think, boy, I didn't work all those years and get a graduate degree to sit around in playgroups in the park."

Like everything else in their structured-for-success lives, the baby, too, was planned, along with the decision for Claudia to return to work after the maximum leave. What wasn't planned, however, was the way she feels now.

"In a way, I don't recognize myself," she says. "It's like I'm a whole different person since the baby's come, with a whole new view of the world. My old life doesn't hold the same allure that it did before, but then again the life of a stay-at-home mom doesn't seem all that exciting either."

On this day at least, Claudia concludes that she'll return to her job next month because she really doesn't have the luxury of choice between working or staying at home full time. Financially, the couple planned to live without her income only temporarily. "Maybe I'll return to work, but I'll change careers," she suggests suddenly. "Now there's another alternative."

Even when they're planned, things don't always work out the way we expected them to. Situations change, people change, and priorities change, and then you have to adapt, together. Claudia's dilemma is common, particularly among bright, high-achieving women who want to do everything right, including parenthood.

But other life changes also can get people sidetracked and cause the reevaluation of career goals: a corporate restructuring or the unexpected loss of a position, a serious illness, a geographic relocation, an unexpected family demand, even a sudden windfall in the form of an inheritance or a spouse's promotion. Just as career demands can fluctuate over a lifetime, so too can the importance we attach to the place of work in our lives, or to the kind of work we do.

Dealing with Change

"Not only are we not on the fast-track," jokes Amit, "I'd say we're actually parked somewhere off on the shoulder of the road!"

Since they were married a year and a half ago, Amit and Maureen have faced lots of changes. First there was the good news: right before the wedding, Amit was awarded a teaching fellowship to pursue his Ph.D. Then there was the bad news: they both had to move away from family and friends, and Maureen had to leave a lucrative job in a city she loved and adjust to life as the wife of a struggling student in a community where little other than academia is going on. She's spent a lot of time alone, and decent jobs have been hard to find. She's just quit her most recent job, in fact, which she hated, without a new position to go to. That makes her husband a little nervous.

"Amit says that I have to be the only Ivy League graduate in the country with zero career ambition," Maureen laughs, "but, seriously, it's okay. I have some vacation pay coming, and I'll do temp work. We'll get by while we're waiting for life to start."

The feeling that "life hasn't started yet" is a common one among couples like Amit and Maureen, couples who are still in school, or still trying to get themselves situated into careers, or still trying to fit into new communities. Not uncommonly, these couples usually have fairly clear long-term goals: Amit, for instance, is pursuing a Ph.D. with the hope of becoming a college professor, a career that is intellectually challenging, but which will also allow him time for his family. Maureen has a solid undergraduate education and fully expects to work most of her life, but she too wants a family, and so her career aspirations are clearly secondary to family goals.

According to the Bureau of Labor Statistics, the average adult changes occupations—not jobs, but occupations—every six and a half years. That works out to an average of four career changes over a 25- to 30-year work life; job changes within the same career are simply too numerous to count. Sometimes these changes are forced, sometimes they're by choice, but either way, a number of personal, financial, and emotional upheavals are to be expected.

Couples deal with these upheavals in different ways and with varying degrees of success. "Generally, people who have just finished school or just relocated or are in some other early part of the process of trying to jump-start their careers usually handle temporary setbacks better than those who think they are established and thus have higher expectations of themselves," says a placement counselor with a large employment agency. (See "Problems of Relocation" in Chapter 1, and "Handling Crises" in Chapter 2.)

Humor helps Amit and Maureen deal with their uncertainties, and they try to remember to enjoy the one thing they know they have—each other. "We don't have much money, and we may not have much job security right now," Maureen says, "but we have time together and we truly enjoy each other. We laugh, and we read, and we exercise, and we shop for bargains. Really, I think a lot of couples our age miss out on the simple pleasure in each other's company that we're enjoying."

"Yeah," Amit agrees. "You know, sometimes when you know you have a long drive ahead of you, it's sort of nice to pull off onto the shoulder of the road and just sit and admire the scenery."

Redefining Your Goals

What seems reasonable, in terms of work schedules and goals, at the very beginning of a marriage doesn't always prove valid over time. Particularly demanding routines have a way of taking over, of becoming larger than the people who live them. Without periodic reevaluation, it's easy to lose sight of why you're living, working, and running the way you do.

Warren and Hilda met in paramedic school. It wasn't easy for them to find time to date, much less time to get married, but they managed in between emergencies. Both high-energy, goal-oriented people, the couple determined what they wanted out of life and set out to achieve it. "Almost from the day we got home from the honeymoon," Hilda says, "we put ourselves to task for our first goal: a home of our own." As incredible as it seems, Warren and Hilda managed to save the down payment, $20,000, in just over a year.

Of course, they each had to work two jobs to do it: Warren as a full-time firefighter and a part-time paramedic, Hilda as a full-time paramedic and part-time doctor's assistant, and both of them teaching Emergency Medical Service courses on the side. "The satisfaction of reaching our goal, of working as a team toward something we both wanted was a real high," Hilda admits. "But once you put yourself on that kind of treadmill, it's hard to get off. It sort of perpetuates itself.

"The goal, and the routines to achieve it, got bigger than we were. We forgot we were people who needed to go to the movies occasionally or have a little fun. We had a house, but we didn't have a life!"

As the tension built and the distance between them grew, they recognized that they had to sit down and "regroup," as Hilda puts it. Their immediate goal of buying a house had long since been achieved, so it was time to take another look at their career choices in light of new, longer-term goals.

"Honestly, I think that even though we got married, we really postponed our marriage to finish up things that we should have done before, such as Warren establishing some financial security and my completing my education," Hilda states frankly. "Those things were important to us before, but we kind of set them aside in the romance of being in love."

It's not uncommon to lose sight of personal goals in the heady experience of falling in love and planning a wedding. It's not even uncommon to supplant personal goals with couple goals, such as Hilda and Warren did with buying a house. But, at some point, the old aspirations will surface once again and, if not attended to, may breed resentment and regret. "Our challenge now is to satisfy our personal goals while also considering each other and the marriage," Hilda explains. "It isn't easy, but at least now we're aware of the challenge and we're working at it. And we know things will get better soon."

The couple still lives what most would consider a dizzying schedule, but for them, there's a focus and an end in sight. Hilda is working part-time at night as a paramedic and finishing up her nursing degree during the day, while Warren rotates between days and nights as a firefighter. Three nights a week the couple is on duty, in the same city, often working together. And they do plan ahead more now and make dates to be together alone or with friends.

The pursuit of a formal education is an important personal goal for Hilda, but also a practical goal for them as a couple. Hilda expects to gain more control over her work schedule as a nurse, and to make more money. Eventually, she would like to get her master's degree and go into teaching. With a better income and a little more time flexibility, Hilda and Warren might be able to relax and enjoy life while also working at professions they consider meaningful and satisfying. "We've even been socking away $20 a week for a second honeymoon when I finish my degree next year," Hilda confides.

High-Anxiety Occupations

As if the rigors of their schedules weren't enough, Warren and Hilda both have chosen high-anxiety occupations as a way of life. Firefighting, emergency services, medicine, law enforcement, and similarly stressful professions place a unique and permanent strain on marriage. Obviously, it's a strain that many couples can't withstand, as evidenced by the proportionately higher divorce rates among those in high-anxiety fields.

What Other Couples Say . . .

Whether it's high-stress professions, such as medicine or law, or high-risk occupations, such as policework or firefighting, the consensus among couples interviewed was that it's easier to handle the job stress when both spouses are in the same or similar occupations. Even though pressures come into the marriage from both partners, the increased level of understanding and identification each brings to the other's situation mitigates some of the negative effects.

As one newlywed stated, "You don't have to explain all the time why you feel the way you do. You just know he understands, and there's unspoken comfort in that."

"Yes, our jobs are important, rewarding, even exciting sometimes," says an emergency-room doctor, "but they can also be frustrating, exhausting, and emotionally draining. Some days you don't have much of yourself left to bring home. Unfortunately, your spouse has to learn to live with that."

That's not always easy to do. Hilda, for instance, feels she's better equipped than most to be the wife of a firefighter because she's a paramedic and so understands the dangers and pressures of Warren's job. Nevertheless, his inability to vent his emotions and share his frustrations at home sometimes creates a communications block between them. "I know what it's like to come home and be angry at the world," she says. "You've seen suffering and pain all day long, so the last thing you want to do is talk more about it or hear about somebody else's problems. I do understand that, but I also know that you can't live totally inside yourself. You can't just shut out those who love you."

Finding the line between being supportive and being intrusive is difficult for every couple at first, but it is especially difficult for those trying to counterbalance a high-stress work life with a low-key home life. Couples in these situations talk a lot about confidence and competence, and about how fear, worry, and additional stress at home can actually undermine one's judgment and performance on the job, thereby increasing whatever risk or anxiety already exists for that partner.

"Basically, when you marry the person, you marry the profession, too," Hilda says, "literally for better or worse. No matter how bizarre or dangerous the profession is, you have to learn to look at it as a job, the same as any other job, so you can establish a normal home life. Otherwise, you won't be able to cope."

Competition or Cooperation?

Most people spend approximately 30 percent of their lives at work. That's a lot of time to spend at an activity you hate, and not enough time to spend at something you love. Keeping your job in proper perspective means finding the right balance between those two poles.

Hating a job presents a peculiar kind of stress, but at least the workday doesn't tend to expand. In contrast, the more you love your work or care about what you do, the more encroaching it's likely to become. Business travel, at-home paperwork, emergency calls, mental preoccupation, corporate entertaining, all valid job-related activities, start to lay claim to the other two-thirds of your life. And though your spouse may understand, even admire, your career commitment, that doesn't mean he or she won't grow to resent your involvement or begin to feel a need to compete for your time and attention.

"If you can't beat 'em, you join 'em," jokes Carol good-naturedly. "Steve's company is not part of our lives, it *is* our lives. To be honest, I knew it would be that way when I married him, so I can't say that's been a surprise." What has been surprising is how Carol has come to deal with the situation by getting extremely involved in the business, too.

Remember Carol and Steve from Chapter 2? They're the couple who lived together for a year to make sure they could manage a relationship in the midst of Steve's fast-paced, entrepreneurial lifestyle. What they've found is that they can not only manage it, they can succeed as partners on all fronts.

"I was in sales for another company," explains Carol, "and then once Steve and I got married, I started to travel with him sometimes, to share his business entertaining, and to help out here and there. And then I thought, this is stupid. Why am I working for somebody else? Is it just to prove my own independence?"

From worrying about the liabilities his work presented to their relationship, Steve gradually began to see what an asset Carol was and how much fun they could have working together. "Maybe I was a little afraid of the competition at first," he admits sheepishly.

For Carol and Steve, a potentially threatening, competitive situation has turned into successful, happy cooperation. They realize that they may have to alter their lifestyle as circumstances change, for instance when children come, but they feel the experience of having established a true partnership, in life and in business, will be an effective preventative against any future conflicts or misunderstandings about the role of work in their lives.

Every couple has to strike this balance between work and family life for themselves and in their own way. Some will do it through mutual identification and equal career participation, as have this couple and the pediatricians and the paramedics we met earlier. Others will find balance through more complementary career choices, seeking to offset one partner's more demanding job with the other's more adaptive situation. Still others will agree that they only "work to live," and so will place more emphasis on other areas of life rather than on their jobs.

It doesn't matter how a couple works out the career choices between them or what they decide, as long as they communicate honestly and openly. Each must strive to reach a true understanding of the role of work in the other's life. Otherwise, conflicts and resentments over career obligations are bound to erupt.

Socrates said that a man is what he does. Certainly, our deeds and accomplishments speak for us, but we also have to speak for ourselves, especially to those we love.

CHAPTER 8

Managing Your Money: Short-Term Solutions

M oney, money, money, money,
Money, money, money, money,
Money, money,
Money, money,
Money, money, money, money.

Sometimes it seems as if money is all people talk about, think about, worry about. It is the undisputed leader as a cause of disagreements among married couples. Part of the preoccupation with this topic is no doubt due to the uncertain financial climate in our country and throughout the world.

Good.

Good?!?!?

Yes, good—particularly for newlyweds. You see, when the economy is booming, everybody, even the government, tends to live like a sailor on a weekend pass. There's no worry about tomorrow, just buy, buy, buy today. That's exactly what happened in the eighties that got us into this financial fix, and that's exactly when American consumers began amassing their own unprecedented level of individual debt, debt that most of us are still struggling to pay off. Sure, it was fun while it lasted, but it was hardly a climate conducive to developing fiscal responsibility.

Now times are tighter, fiscal policies are more conservative, and consumers are more cautious. People are more conscious of their own spending habits. An atmosphere of restraint and responsibility prevails, and that atmosphere *is* conducive to fostering the kind of reasonable, intelligent earning and spending habits you as newlyweds must cultivate in order to establish a sound financial partnership from the very beginning.

Money Messages

"Some of my earliest memories are of my parents fighting over money," Terry recalls. "They fought about it all the time. Then, when I was 12, they got a di-

---

❧❧   DO YOU SEE YOURSELF HERE?   ❧❧

- Do the two of you come from different socioeconomic backgrounds?
- Has marriage dramatically altered the lifestyle for one of you?
- Have you found yourselves in conflict over differences in your attitudes toward money or your money-management styles?
- Have you had difficulty agreeing on the division of financial chores and responsibilities?
- Do you argue over the personal spending habits of one partner?
- Do you find it difficult to talk about money?
- Did one or both of you come to the marriage with considerable debt?
- Do you disagree over the use of credit?
- Are you living from paycheck to paycheck, operating without a household budget?
- Are you unable to save regularly?
- Are you basically spending everything you make?

Read on to solve the dilemmas indicated by "yes" answers.

---

vorce, but they still fought about money because my mother always said we didn't have enough. Personally, I hate to talk about money, so I don't. The subject is too depressing."

Most of us may not have the dramatic childhood associations with money that Terry has, but we do come to marriage with certain attitudes and associations in place, some that we may not even be aware of. These attitudes reflect our family backgrounds and the ways we experienced money being used, or abused, while growing up.

While most families don't openly discuss their finances around the dinner table, at least not with the children, it's still pretty easy for a youngster to see how money affects the behavior of parents and other adult relatives. Eventually, the child falls heir to a collective family attitude toward what money represents. Thus, we come to see it as a symbol of love, power, or security, and we come to believe either that "money is the root of all evil" or that "you can never be too rich or too thin." (Actually, most of us vacillate and probably believe a little bit of both.)

As members of a family, children don't make lifestyle choices; they inherit them. Consequently, one's economic condition, be it hardship or affluence, and the pressures or privileges that go along with it, are largely taken for granted. Unless there is some pointed reason to call the habits of that lifestyle into question, the values and behaviors it inculcates are likely to continue into adulthood.

This means that we have to be realistic about our own past experience and understand the hang-ups or limitations our backgrounds might have imposed. For instance, if a child grows up dining in fine restaurants, summering in the Hamptons, and saying "I'll take it" before she's even looked at the price tag, it's going to be hard for her to understand the value of a dollar, or to learn to live on a limited budget. On the other hand, if material wealth was used as a substitute for love and attention in her home, then she may come to resent or distrust money, rebel against her social class, and adopt an adult lifestyle that is not only different, but perhaps downright austere.

The psychology of money is a complicated matter, indeed, as any successful salesperson or advertising executive can tell you. Unless they have so much that they don't even have to think about it, most people do not have neutral, totally objective attitudes about financial matters. Rather, they bring their subliminal associations, their personal financial habits, and sometimes their visceral reactions, along with them to any monetary discussion. Or, like Terry, they refuse to discuss it at all.

It's best if you don't take a position of avoidance with your spouse where your financial partnership is concerned. Try to be as objective as you can in assessing the effects of your own family background and personal financial history, and own up to your fears, fantasies, and fetishes about money. By anticipating and defusing issues that could be potentially explosive between you, you'll begin to establish the kind of forethought, consideration, and communication so essential to successful financial planning.

Do You Have a Money-Management Style?

Newlyweds come to marriage with financial habits they don't even think about, and then are amazed to find that their partner behaves in a different way in the same situation. That's how conflict begins.

Don't fight about your differences, laugh about them. Take this little inventory just for fun, so you'll be sure to keep on laughing—all the way to the bank. Each of you should record your answers separately, and then compare.

1. When I see something I like in a store, I'm likely to say
   a. charge it!
   b. I'll think about it.
   c. I don't really need that.
2. I enjoy money most when
   a. spending it on others.
   b. I'm able to buy something I have been saving for.
   c. I know I have a nice, secure bank balance.
3. I enjoy money least when I
   a. have to worry about it.
   b. have to talk about it.
   c. have to pay bills and taxes.
4. If I won the lottery tomorrow, I'd
   a. have a heck of a good time!
   b. take care of my family, give some to charity, but also enjoy life a little.
   c. invest most of it and make it grow.

5. Money may not be able to buy happiness,
   a. but I'd rather be unhappy with it than without it.
   b. and there are more important things in life anyway.
   c. but not having any guarantees unhappiness.
6. My usual method of bill paying is
   a. to ignore them and see if they'll go away.
   b. to "play the float" and use the grace period.
   c. to pay them promptly when they arrive.
7. My mother always told me
   a. I'd better marry someone rich.
   b. hard work is not always rewarded in this life.
   c. be independent and learn to take care of yourself.
8. To me, a good investment opportunity is
   a. wearable art.
   b. a house.
   c. a diversified portfolio of stocks, bonds, and mutual funds.
9. When it comes to credit card debt,
   a. I'm trying to stage a leveraged buyout!
   b. I get nervous.
   c. I pay cash and don't believe in credit.
10. The last savings deposit I made was
    a. into my piggy bank when I was nine years old.
    b. through the payroll deduction plan at work.
    c. sizable.
11. If I were strapped for cash, I'd
    a. use credit or call my mom.
    b. consider taking on a second job.
    c. be certain that the bank or the accountant had made an error.
12. "Penny wise and pound foolish" means
    a. spending money for a diet program that doesn't work.
    b. driving all over town just to save a dollar or two.
    c. nothing; a penny saved is always a penny earned.
13. The money-management skill that I'm most proud of is
    a. my ability to shop without guilt.
    b. my ability to stretch a budget and live within my means.
    c. my ability to accrue more wealth than my income would seem to allow.

Scoring: Give yourself 3 points for every "a" answer, 2 points for every "b," and 1 point for each "c." Then total your column and refer below.

29 to 36 points—Born to Be Rich
You don't have a money-management style, but you have a great sense of humor. You probably have a wonderful wardrobe, too, and your friends have probably gotten lots of postcards from exotic vacation spots. But, we all know that you've spent every dime you've made since you got out of school and that you don't have much more than memories to show for it.

You really need to work on developing some fiscal responsibility. Why don't you take a night course? And, please, resist the temptation to charge the tuition on your credit card!

21 to 28 points—Born to Be Trusted

You're the salt of the earth, the backbone of the nation, the reasonable, rational, dependable middle-class citizen. Not only do you work hard to cultivate and maintain a responsible money-management style, but you worry about your bills and sincerely try to keep up. You want to believe that others are as honest and reliable as you are.

You could stand to loosen up a little and pat yourself on the back. Why don't you take yourself and your beloved out to a romantic dinner, and charge it—just this once.

12 to 20 points—Born to Be Dull

You could stand to loosen up a lot! And you could start by releasing that death grip you've got on the savings account.

Your diligence and discipline are admirable, but your rigid money-management style is hard for others to live with, especially when you fail to find the humor in overdrafts. Be daring; do something reckless. Buy a Harley or vacation in Tahiti—or both!

Mergers and Acquisitions

It doesn't matter how long you've known each other or how much in love you are, no two people are going to think and behave exactly alike when it comes to money matters. Whatever your individual backgrounds and money-management styles, you must find a way to merge them into a workable system that will not only ensure a firm financial footing for you as a couple, but will also keep you happy and compatible as partners.

"Two people couldn't be more diverse in their spending habits than David and I," says Emily. "Before we were married, I spent every dime I made on clothes and eating out, and he lived like a hermit as a graduate student."

"Yeah, and since we've been married, my standard of living has increased dramatically, and Emily's has plummeted," David laughs. "Seriously, though, we're both trying to move toward the middle in our attitudes."

Even if your spending habits aren't as wildly divergent as Emily's and David's, you'll still have to make adjustments and "move toward the middle" in combining your attitudes. And, it'll help if you have their sense of humor about doing it, because partnership does not mean that one partner's style automatically dominates; rather, for you both to be committed to your financial plan, you each have to contribute to shaping it and making the decisions. That means you're each going to have to compromise in order to establish money-management methods that are comfortable for both of you.

Karen Spero, a certified financial planner and chair of Spero Financial Services, Inc., in Cleveland, has been helping engaged and newlywed couples set up financial housekeeping for over 20 years. "Every choice to spend or save

---

What Other Couples Say . . .

Year after year, in study after study, money continues to rank first as the most common, most universal source of ongoing conflict in marriage. A *Modern Bride* Consumer Council Survey (Cahners, July 1993) substantiated those findings even among newlywed couples, with 50 percent of respondents citing money as the most common cause of contention between them.

---

is unique," she says. "The choice reflects a person's individual values, background, and experience. It isn't really a matter of an attitude being right or wrong; it's a matter of what works in a given situation."

Financial advisers and marriage counselors all can tell harrowing stories of couples married 20, 30, even 40 years or more who still argue about the bills each month. They can't have financial discussions without extreme hostility; they hide purchases from each other or use buying and spending to get even; and they continue, even in their older years, to find new ways to sabotage financial cooperation.

None of this has to be true for the two of you, but you must assess where you've been before you can determine where you're going. "It's often very difficult to identify past discretionary spending patterns," Spero says. "All you know is you don't have any money left, and you're not entirely sure why. That admission, alone, can be a painful and embarrassing process, and many couples find they need a catalyst, a third-party professional, to help them do it."

"However it's done, though," she continues, "a married couple must cultivate the habit of full disclosure in their financial discussions with each other, and they must learn to communicate without angry accusations and harsh judgments. Only then can they hope to manage their partnership smoothly and effectively, and to survive the financial sandtraps that lie between them and their goals."

The Bottom Line

Experts agree that you start your financial assessment by tallying up what you have (assets) and what you owe (liabilities). This tabulation is called "figuring your net worth," and nothing will show you where you stand at a glance better than this exercise. If you've done a net worth statement before, it may be time to do it again and compare where you were then with where you are now. But, if you haven't ever done this before, there's no time like the present.

So, put on a pot of coffee or tea, turn on the answering machine, and settle yourselves in at the dining room table (if you have one!). You will need the following records to complete this exercise:

• Your income tax returns for the last couple of years, or for however long you've been working

- Current bank statements, including checking, savings, trust funds, CDs, etc.
- Other investment statements, such as those from brokerage houses, mutual funds, employee benefit and retirement plans, etc.
- Current payroll stubs
- Insurance policies and statements of cash values
- Personal property records, to help ascertain the value of major items such as jewelry, cars, artwork, collections, real estate, silver, antiques, etc.
- Loan agreements, including mortgage, car loan or lease, college loan, etc.
- Current consumer charge account statements, including store charges and bank credit cards

Now begin to fill in the form that follows. Whatever you can't substantiate with your records, estimate as closely as possible. It's not so important that these figures be exact as it is that the two of you are honest with yourselves and each other.

The following net worth exercise will give you a quick picture of where you are right now. If you see, for instance, that your yearly expenses are *more than* your yearly income, you'll know that you have to get serious about monitoring your spending habits and bringing your budget in line. And, if your total liabilities are more than your total assets, your first priority absolutely has to be to reduce some of that debt.

Your Net Worth Statement

Date Prepared:

	His	Hers	Ours	Total
INCOME (gross)				
Wages	_____	_____	_____	_____
Bonuses	_____	_____	_____	_____
Interest Income	_____	_____	_____	_____
Other	_____	_____	_____	_____
Total Income				_____
EXPENSES (yearly)				
Taxes (federal/state)	_____	_____	_____	_____
Social Security	_____	_____	_____	_____
Other taxes	_____	_____	_____	_____
Mortgage/rent	_____	_____	_____	_____
Real estate tax	_____	_____	_____	_____
Utilities	_____	_____	_____	_____
Car loan/lease payments	_____	_____	_____	_____
Other loan payments	_____	_____	_____	_____
Transportation (gas/commute)	_____	_____	_____	_____
Food	_____	_____	_____	_____
Clothing	_____	_____	_____	_____
Insurance premiums				
Life	_____	_____	_____	_____
Auto	_____	_____	_____	_____

(continued)

Homeowner's   _____ _____ _____ _____
Other   _____ _____ _____ _____
Savings/investments   _____ _____ _____ _____
Pension plans   _____ _____ _____ _____
Medical   _____ _____ _____ _____
Credit card payments   _____ _____ _____ _____
Child care   _____ _____ _____ _____
Child support/alimony   _____ _____ _____ _____
Miscellaneous   _____ _____ _____ _____
     Total Expenses   _____

ASSETS

Cash
   Checking accounts   _____ _____ _____ _____

   Savings accounts   _____ _____ _____ _____

   Money market/CDs/Treasury/Bonds _____ _____ _____ _____
   _____ _____ _____ _____
   _____ _____ _____ _____

     Total Cash   _____
Cash value investments
Brokerage accounts   _____ _____ _____
   _____ _____ _____

401K/IRA/Keogh   _____ _____ _____ _____
   _____ _____ _____ _____

Profit sharing/pensions   _____ _____ _____ _____
Cash value life insurance   _____ _____ _____ _____
Other   _____ _____ _____ _____
     Total Cash Value   _____
Personal property★
   Home/condo   _____ _____ _____ _____
   Other real estate   _____ _____ _____ _____
   Cars   _____ _____ _____ _____
   Jewelry/furs/silver   _____ _____ _____ _____
   Art/antiques/collections   _____ _____ _____ _____
   Furnishings   _____ _____ _____ _____
   Other   _____ _____ _____ _____
     Total Property   _____
     Total Assets   _____

LIABILITIES

Total mortgage   _____ _____ _____ _____
Other loans   _____ _____ _____ _____
Total consumer debt   _____ _____ _____ _____
     Total Liabilities   _____

NET WORTH (Assets minus liabilities)   _____

★Estimate the worth of personal property for its resale value, not what you paid for it.

Developing a Plan

Think of marriage as a business; the idea is for your partnership to be financially profitable. You want to do more than just stay one step ahead of creditors; you want to thrive and flourish so you can turn your future dreams into reality, and the two of you can achieve a reasonable measure of financial security and independence.

The most fundamental principle of good money management is just common sense: you have to spend less than you make. It's that simple, and that difficult. If you don't learn to do that, you'll not only live with constant short-term money worries, but you'll get farther and farther away from your long-term goals.

Devising a workable financial plan, then, involves both the skillful management of day-to-day cash flow, usually achieved through a household budget, and the mutual agreement on long-term financial goals, from which short-term spending priorities are determined. In the beginning, however, putting a plan together is a little bit like asking, "Which comes first, the chicken or the egg?" You can't really set long-term goals until you get on top of your cash flow, but you can't set spending priorities until you have some long-term goals. Where do you start?

You've already begun when you sat down and completed the net worth statement. From that you can get at least a preliminary indication of what your overall financial picture looks like. Then, to this, you should add an honest appraisal of your particular spending habits and choices. Here are some questions for analysis and discussion between the two of you:

- Are you living under a cloud of inordinate debt: home loans, car loans, student loans, maxed-out credit cards? If so, maybe getting out from under that should be your first goal, particularly from the short-term, high-interest debt like that on bank credit cards.
- Does either of you have a troubled credit history? Have you declared bankruptcy, resorted to consolidation loans, or used one credit source to pay off another? Is one of you likely to be negatively affected by the credit history of the other? If so, perhaps you should consider keeping your affairs separate, at least for a while, with bank accounts, credit cards, and even income taxes under each name.
- Are you spending money for things that don't turn into assets, such as high monthly rent, fancy car leases, or rentals on furniture or other equipment? Might it be time to reevaluate some of those lifestyle choices? True, you might have to live with less, but at least you'll own what you have.
- Do you eat out frequently or buy gourmet takeout, spend large sums of money for auxiliary services (laundry and dry cleaning, housekeeping, beauty salon, cable TV, etc.), or fail to take advantage of sales and coupons because shopping where you shop is more convenient? It's incredible how much money just slips through our fingers. On a typical Saturday morning, for instance, you might make a stop at the corner grocer, the dry cleaner's, the drugstore, the shoe repair, the barber shop, and bam! $100 is gone. Go out for a nice dinner on a Saturday night, and you're on your way to a $200 weekend.

- Have you been saving at all? Even as little as $50 a month, given dollar cost averaging in a mutual fund, can add up. Saving doesn't have to be dramatic, but it does have to be regular. Every financial expert says the same thing: pay yourselves first!
- How much do you know about handling money and managing investments? For all of our education, financial experts agree that there is a deplorable ignorance on the part of otherwise intelligent, well-educated people about financial matters. Many banks and brokerage houses give free clinics and seminars, and courses on various aspects of money management are routinely offered in night school and through the continuing education divisions of community colleges and universities. Take advantage of the offerings in your area. It's something the two of you can do together that is in your own best interest.

The Household Budget

Now that you've ascertained your assets and liabilities (net worth) and begun to compare your attitudes and analyze your spending habits, the two of you are ready to devise a cash flow plan, which most people call a household budget.

Thanks to the American Institute of Certified Public Accountants, we were able to engage the professional services of Lyle K. Benson, Jr., a partner in the Baltimore accounting firm of Coyne & McClean Chartered, to construct a sample cash flow statement for a newlywed couple. He used a combined yearly gross income of $54,200, which was the average newlywed income among those surveyed in a *Modern Bride* Consumer Council Study (Cahners, July 1993).

While this budget is hypothetical and makes some assumptions about how our "average" couple lives, the way it is constructed and the guidelines a certified public accountant and certified financial planner used to do it should be helpful to you in structuring your own cash flow plan. Study the categories and disbursements of the *Modern Bride* couple first, paying particular attention to the way their income is distributed. The percentages can be useful guidelines, but they should not be interpreted as rigid rules. After you've examined the sample, you can then copy the blank form and adjust it for structuring your own household budget.

"The most important element of planning your cash flow is to prepare a realistic budget and stick to it," Lyle Benson says. "There are many ways to track the budget, depending on how detailed you want to be, but the most important purpose is to help you live within your means so you can reach the financial goals you've set."

Benson cautions couples to be particularly mindful of the miscellaneous cash category, what he calls the "mystery hole" into which so many well-intentioned budgets fall. "You have to know where your dollars are going," he says. "By tracking cash advances from ATM machines, checks written to cash, and other out-of-pocket expenditures, you will be able to see how much of your money is going toward unidentified expenses. Then you may be able to identify them."

Sample Cash Flow Statement
(For Financial Planning Purposes Only)

	AMOUNT (yearly)	AMOUNT (monthly)	PERCENT (of net)
Sources of Cash:			
Gross salaries	$54,200		
Dividend/interest			
Sales of securities			
Business income			
Rental income			
Other income			
Total Source of Cash	$54,200		
Income Taxes:			
Federal	5,260		
State	2,993		
FICA	4,146		
Net Income	$41,861	$3,488	100%
Uses of Cash:			
Savings and investments	4,000	333	10%
Fixed outflows:			
Mortgage note payments★	9,478	790	23%
Other insurance premiums	2,206	184	5%
Other note payments			
Total Fixed Outflow	15,684	1,307	38%
Variable Outflows:			
Food	6,000	500	14%
Transportation (car payments, etc.)	6,000	500	14%
Utilities	3,000	250	7%
Clothes/personal care	3,600	250	9%
Recreation/vacation	2,000	167	5%
Medical/dental	1,000	82	2%
Donations	600	33	1%
Property taxes	1,500	125	4%
Other taxes			
Education			
Entertainment	1,200	100	3%
Miscellaneous	1,200	100	3%
Total Variable Outflows	$26,100	2,175	62%
Total All Uses of Cash	$41,784	3,482	100%
Total Expenses	$54,123		
Net Profit/Loss	+ $ 77		

★Based on home mortgage of $100,000 @ 8½% for 30 years; includes yearly interest ($8,400), principal ($828), and homeowners' insurance ($250).

Your Cash Flow Statement
(For Financial Planning Purposes Only)

	AMOUNT (yearly)	AMOUNT (monthly)	PERCENT (of net)
Sources of Cash:			
Gross salaries	_____	_____	_____
Dividend/interest	_____	_____	_____
Sales of securities	_____	_____	_____
Business income	_____	_____	_____
Rental income	_____	_____	_____
Other income	_____	_____	_____
Total Source of Cash	_____	_____	_____
Income Taxes:			
Federal	_____	_____	_____
State	_____	_____	_____
FICA	_____	_____	_____
Net Income	_____	_____	_____
Uses of Cash:			
Savings and investments	_____	_____	_____
Fixed outflows:			
Mortgage note payments	_____	_____	_____
Other insurance premiums	_____	_____	_____
Other note payments			
Total Fixed Outflow	_____	_____	_____
Variable Outflows:			
Food	_____	_____	_____
Transportation (car payments, etc.)	_____	_____	_____
Utilities	_____	_____	_____
Clothes/personal care	_____	_____	_____
Recreation/vacation	_____	_____	_____
Medical/dental	_____	_____	_____
Donations	_____	_____	_____
Property taxes	_____	_____	_____
Other taxes	_____	_____	_____
Education	_____	_____	_____
Entertainment	_____	_____	_____
Miscellaneous	_____	_____	_____
Total Variable Outflows	_____	_____	_____
Total All Uses of Cash	_____	_____	_____
Total Expenses	_____		
Net Profit/Loss	_____		

Dividing the Money-Management Tasks

Here is a list of what you have to do to keep your financial partnership in working order:

- Be employed.
- Manage the cash flow on your monthly budget.
- Keep records for yourselves and the IRS.
- Monitor intermediate savings and investments for emergency reserves and for particular purchases.
- Control debt by keeping track of charge cards and short-term consumer interest.
- Plan for taxes. April rolls around quickly; ideally tax planning should take place all year long.
- Keep track of insurance policies and benefits, including filing claims and recording reimbursements.
- Manage long-term investments, including estate planning and retirement.

It takes a lot of work to keep one's financial affairs in order, to stay informed, and to make wise saving and spending choices. Obviously, some of these tasks are more time-consuming than others, and some tasks are regular and some periodic. But, as you can see, there's more than enough here for both of you to do to feel needed, useful, and actively involved in your combined financial decisions. And it all works best if you both are actively involved!

As married partners, you are both responsible for your financial affairs under the law, so you should both be responsible at home, too. Neither of you can afford to be ignorant about your own affairs, or ignorant about money matters in general—not in this economy. There is a lot to do to manage a household, more, realistically speaking, than one of you should have to do alone. Each of you has skills and talents to contribute. If you don't, it's time you develop some.

Here are some basic management suggestions:

- Divide the list of tasks on the basis of preference, time, and aptitude. The one who likes to study up and research long-term issues might be suited to taking responsibility for record keeping, investments, and taxes, while the other would assume responsibility for short-term chores. Or, if you have lots of evenings at home together, you can both do everything, including bill paying, together. Regardless of who does what, make sure your records are organized so that either spouse can easily find information.
- Establish and/or maintain some credit accounts in your own name, not as "Mrs. John Smith," and not as a second cardholder on your spouse's account. Both men and women need to establish their own independent credit histories. (See more about credit vs. cash later in this chapter, and more about women and credit history in Chapter 10.)
- Consider having three checking accounts: yours, mine, and ours. For the sake of privacy and independence, each of you needs to have your own money to spend as you like without your partner's knowledge or consent,

even if it's only a small amount. But, you also need a household account into which you each contribute a certain percentage of your paychecks, and out of which bills, taxes, and common expenses are paid. (If you do have separate accounts, be sure that your partner has his or her signature registered at the bank so, in the event of your illness or demise, your spouse could have access to those funds. Otherwise, they would be frozen. Joint accounts, checking or savings, should read "Mary Smith *or* John Smith," not "and." "And" requires both signatures.)

- Many couples do share just one common checking account, but record keeping can be harrowing in that arrangement, especially if your spending styles are different. Other couples each have separate accounts, and then agree between them who will pay what household expense. That's okay, as long as you don't argue about who's paying a greater percentage of common expenses. Ultimately, the choice is whatever works for you, but a strong argument is being made here for each of you to have some discretionary funds and individual credit cards, and therefore some financial freedom, of your own.

- If you have a home computer, consider one of the excellent (and very reasonably priced) personal financial management software programs. The best of them will not only monitor the household budget, keep track of personal checkbooks, and actually print checks or transfer funds electronically for paying bills, but they can also record expenditures by category for income tax purposes and track investments, including simple mutual fund or stock portfolios. Using such programs will also teach you more about money management.

- It's never too early to begin tax planning, starting with an analysis of last year's tax returns (for each of you or the two of you together). Make sure that your withholdings or estimated payments were sufficient so that there are no surprises this year, and no penalties. If you are self-employed, remember that the self-employment tax takes a big chunk out of your budget on a quarterly basis, which should be planned for in the budget. (See more about taxes in Chapter 9.)

Making a Budget Work

"We keep redoing the budget, and redoing the budget," laments one newlywed. "No matter how we do it, things always look great on paper, but never work out in real life."

"A budget must be flexible in order to work," says Benson, "and it has to be reevaluated regularly in light of changing circumstances and new information. Interest rates change, tax laws change, you get a raise—even deciding you need a new winter coat can necessitate alterations in the budget."

There are three kinds of expenses: **fixed,** those that stay the same every month for a long period of time, such as your rent or mortgage or a car payment; **periodic,** those that are predictable amounts and come due regularly, although not monthly, such as property taxes and insurance premiums; and **variable,** those that change depending on need and spending habits, such as groceries, clothing, and entertainment. Obviously, without making a major decision like changing your residence or finding a new insurance carrier, the only expenses you can really monitor and control on a month-to-month basis are the variable ones.

"Yeah, well, but we have to eat," you might say, and that's true enough, but you can alter the way you eat and what you eat. Many of the variable expenses—food, clothing, entertainment, gift giving, hobbies, personal grooming—are matters of taste and style. You may not want to adjust them up or down, but they can be adjusted, or sometimes eliminated entirely, especially when other financial priorities have to come first.

Variable expenses comprise the lion's share of most household budgets and, unless you're living way beyond your means in terms of big houses and fancy cars, the variables are most often to blame when a budget gets out of whack. Too many clothes, too many dinners out, too many getaway weekends and there's sure to be little or nothing left to save.

For most couples, then, balancing a budget means keeping records of your discretionary spending habits, finding out where the money goes, and taking a good look at just how much of it generally goes there. Simple awareness is the first key; making conscious choices about spending is the next one. Financial experts agree that, psychologically, people are more likely to stay within their budgets if they trim variable expenses across the board, often in ways that are hardly noticeable, rather than eliminating some favorite frills altogether. Think of it like dieting: if you say, "I'll never have another piece of chocolate cake again," you're destined to fail before you even begin.

If your income far exceeds your expenses and your budget is working just fine, thank you, then you can ignore this whole discussion. But, if you're like most couples, newlyweds and "olderweds" alike, you're always eager to find painless ways to save.

Ideas for Trimming the Variables

Food

- Use grocery store and drugstore coupons. You don't have to go crazy with this by getting a file and keeping track of rebates; just clipping the coupons in the Sunday paper and using them promptly will save you a few dollars a week. And a few dollars will buy you a nice deli sandwich.
- Don't automatically reach for name brands just because your mother always used them. Check out the generics. If you really don't care about the virtues of a particular product, then don't spend more for it out of habit.
- Don't automatically assume that the larger size is a better value. Often it isn't. True, checking labels and comparing cost and weight takes time, but doing it once should be enough to inform you of what's what.
- You pay for convenience: gourmet takeout, frozen foods, fruits and vegetables already cleaned and chopped. On the other hand, sometimes buying an already-prepared fresh fruit salad for the two of you makes more sense than

buying all the individual fruits and melons it would take to make one. Think about cost effectiveness when you shop.

- Don't grocery shop when you're hungry, and don't shop when you're harassed. Plan your menus in advance, and go to the store with a list in hand. You'll spend less—guaranteed.
- Working couples spend an enormous amount of money eating out, not so much for pleasure and entertainment as just to avoid the chore of cooking. Try these solutions to this problem:
  - Make double recipes of casseroles, spaghetti sauce, etc., to freeze, so all you have to do in the evening is pop the dish in the oven.
  - Go out to lunch or have a hot lunch in your company cafeteria, so you will be satisfied with just a salad or something light for dinner.
  - Plan menus in advance and post the plan on the refrigerator. That way, you'll always know "what's for dinner," and you won't end up "too tired to think about it."
  - Don't be shy about bringing home doggie bags from restaurants to reheat and have another night. While you're at it, if there are specials being offered the night you eat out, something like "buy one pizza, get the second at half price," take advantage of it and take the second one home.
  - Instead of going out for dinner, go out for coffee and dessert.

Clothing

- Adult clothing costs offer big ways to save because purchases can be postponed, sales can be frequented, and bargains can be found. Almost nobody pays full price for anything anymore. Why should you?
- Resist impulse buying and don't stroll the mall just because you're bored. Unless you're window shopping when the stores are closed, "just looking" is bound to cost you something, at least that's what retailers hope. Shopping has become entertainment in our culture, and it's costing us—big time!
- Update your wardrobe twice a year, for the fall/winter, and the spring/ summer. Take an inventory of what you have and what you need, and set a dollar limit, in advance, on what you'll spend. Systematic seasonal shopping has three advantages: everything you buy will coordinate with what you already own; it's easier to control clothing costs when you don't shop often; and you'll save time, as well as money, in the long run.
- Think about the maintenance costs of clothes before you buy them. Garments that must be dry cleaned or otherwise specially treated and handled (such as suedes and leathers) to look good, or items that are fragile (delicate lace, beading, etc.) and will need constant repair, or anything that must be altered or hemmed by a professional (because you don't sew) end up costing more than just the original purchase price.
- Buy accessories, a scarf, belt, or hat, when you feel the need to freshen a tired look and give yourself a lift.
- If you sew, even a little, and you like it, think about investing in some lessons to learn to sew better. Classes, books, and even great home-sewing videos are available to help you. Sewing is a relaxing, satisfying hobby that can save

you an enormous amount of money, and even help you make money if you do it well enough.

Other Incidentals

- Shop around for the best deal on checking and savings accounts. Check charges and monthly fees can add up fast, often when you're not even aware of it. Make the banks compete for your business and look for accounts that offer free or low-fee checking, and that pay interest on your checking account.
- Ditto for phone service. Compare the rates for long-distance carriers, and find out about all the discounts available on calling rates, customer services, and rental equipment from your local phone company. If you have relocated far away from friends and family, higher phone bills may be more of a necessity than a luxury for you. That's understandable, but put a time limit on those regular long-distance calls, so you can budget and anticipate these expenses. Also, investigate price breaks for regularly called area codes.
- For thoughtful, generous people who have large families and many friends, gift-giving is a real budget blower, especially at Christmastime. Try these strategies for controlling costs:
  - Give several small (and less expensive) gifts rather than one big (expensive) one. It will seem like more simply because there's more to open.
  - Buy boxes of greeting cards. They're cheaper that way, and you'll have them on hand when you need them.
  - Call a faraway loved one instead of sending a gift. They'd really rather talk to you than have a present.
  - Shop for those on your gift list all year long, especially for Christmas or Hanukkah. When you see something that's just right for a particular person, pick it up, especially if it's on sale! Doing this helps you avoid the last-minute, I'll-pay-anything method of shopping, and allows you to spread your gift-giving expenses out over a long period of time.
- Look for rebate offers when buying home appliances, and save all warranties for the products you buy. If something breaks or is found to be faulty, the manufacturer's guarantee can save you repair or replacement costs.
- Always check the weekend edition of your local paper for entertaining things to do that don't cost much money. Most communities have something going on that's free or available for nominal cost: garden shows, crafts fairs, open-air concerts, historical exhibits, etc. Invite your friends, have fun, and learn more about where you live.

Cash versus Credit

Ever notice how some people can tell you down to the dollar exactly how much money they have in their wallets at any given moment, whereas others don't even know which pocket or purse their wallet is in, much less if there's anything in it? Is a certain financial acumen just inborn in some people?

Admittedly, it's hard for anybody to keep track of cash, and that's what prompts many to rely on credit cards, at least initially. But then, of course, when you start to lose track of the charge slips, too, you're in big trouble.

"I was one of those people who could never fill a piggy bank as a child, because I was always taking out what I had just put in," Emily confesses. "I'm no good with cash. And now I find myself married to somebody who's accustomed to relying almost totally on cash and using credit cards very little."

But Emily is trying. For example, in order for David to feel secure and to know that they always have ready cash for routine expenses, the couple has created a set of envelopes marked "groceries," "gas," "gifts/entertainment," etc. Each paycheck, a budgeted amount of cash is put into these envelopes. That way, the money is always available, but the couple can also see at a glance if they're staying within their budgetary allowance.

"It works, it really does, as long as I don't go in and raid the envelopes." She laughs. "No, really. I am getting a better sense of cash with this system, and it is nice to know that the money's there for the paperboy, or for a pizza on Friday night."

In the couple's "move toward the middle" ground of their money-management styles, David is also learning something about credit. The two have agreed that certain items, clothing chief among them, will be routinely charged so they'll have records and can begin to track these expenses. "Plus, I do see the advantage of building a positive credit history for the future," he says.

"A lot of spending habits people develop are just that—habits," says Don Badders, president of the nonprofit Consumer Credit Counseling Service. "The habits are developed early on, but they need to change to adapt to new situations. The cash vs. credit controversy is really nothing more than a mindset people have gotten into. It's not an either/or situation; sound financial management involves the judicious use of both."

The Consumer Credit Counseling Service has over 850 offices in the United States, Canada, and Puerto Rico, all of which offer free or low-cost professional financial counseling and debt management (see Appendix for resource). While you don't have to be in serious financial trouble to seek counseling, many people are. "We see couples from all walks of life and from all socioeconomic levels," says Badders. "Money-management skill has nothing to do with income level, or social sophistication, or formal educational background. It's not something you're just born with; it's something you're motivated to learn."

Money Professionals

You don't have to be wealthy to take advantage of the services of a financial professional and, for some couples, especially those who can't seem to get on top of their affairs, the help of an expert may be their only salvation for solvency. Most couples, though, will deal with one or more of these professionals on their way to financial security.

You choose a fiscal adviser based on the kind of help you need. We've already talked about counseling services for debt management, for instance, but

Consumer Credit Counseling Service Debt Test

Debt problems develop over a period of time, and consumers are often unaware they are in serious trouble until it's too late. The National Foundation for Consumer Credit and Consumer Credit Counseling Service have formulated the following test to help consumers know if they should be concerned. If you answer "yes" to two or more of these questions, you need to seek debt counseling.

1. Are you borrowing to pay for items you used to pay for with cash?
2. Is an increasing percentage of your income going to pay off debts?
3. Is your savings cushion inadequate or nonexistent?
4. Can you only make the minimum payments on your revolving charge accounts?
5. Are your lines of credit at or near the limit on your credit cards?
6. Have circumstances forced you to take out a loan to make payments on a previous loan?
7. Are you unsure about how much you owe?
8. Are your monthly credit bills more than 20 percent of your take-home pay (excluding rent or mortgage payments)?
9. If you lost your job, would you be in immediate financial difficulty?

there are all sorts of other services available. Word-of-mouth recommendations from people whose needs and circumstances are similar to your own are the best vehicle for finding a suitable professional, but you can also call industry associations (resources are listed in the Appendix) for referrals where you live.

Make interview appointments with two or three targeted professionals and meet them face to face (see Appendix for interview guidelines offered by the International Association for Financial Planning). There should be no charge for this preliminary interview. Find out about the professional's certifications, specialties, and experience, particularly whether or not they are accustomed to working with younger couples. The professional should seem interested in meeting your needs, and should make the two of you feel comfortable. He or she might even "interview" you in terms of trying to find out more about your money-management experience and the kinds of professional services you may have used before, or are using now.

Here is a brief overview of the kinds of professionals out there and what they can do:

Bankers: It pays to begin establishing a relationship with your bank from the very beginning, even when you're only setting up checking and savings accounts, because your neighborhood banker can be a very good friend to have. Most couples get involved with a bank officer when negotiating a loan or a mortgage, or perhaps when making an investment into a bank money market fund or CD, but increasingly, banks are offering a full range of investment/money-management services. It makes sense to learn how to use the available expertise bankers offer as routine services for their regular customers. There is no charge for a banker's advice, although there may be filing fees for loans and transactional charges for investments.

Accountants (Usually, Certified Public Accountants, see Appendix): While some accountants specialize, most accountants are generalists in tax laws and the effects those laws have on individuals and businesses. Some are also financial planners. If you are self-employed or in business together, or anticipate particular tax complications, or simply need to set up a solid accounting procedure for managing your affairs, an accountant would be helpful. Accountants charge hourly fees, and you should find out in advance what they are.

Financial Planners: They should be certified through one of the major educational designations, which means that they have taken a specialized course of study and worked a minimum number of years in the field (see Appendix). Financial planners concentrate on the big picture, on helping you reach intermediate and long-term financial goals, even to building wealth. To do that, they will first analyze your present financial situation, then show you what steps to take toward your goals, and then help you buy and sell investments (most planners do sell stocks, bonds, mutual funds, etc.). Fees can vary widely, from hourly rates to commissions to a combination of both. Make sure you understand the fee structure before you begin.

Lawyers: Lawyers specialize in various kinds of transactions: taxes, real estate, contracts, trusts and estates, etc. You will need a lawyer on occasion, whenever you are entering into a legal transaction, such as buying a house or drawing up a will, but you would not go to a lawyer for regular financial advice unless your affairs were of such a magnitude that the attorney had been retained to manage them. Lawyers never work on commission; they charge an hourly rate or a flat fee for a particular transaction.

Stockbrokers: A broker is someone who is licensed by the Securities and Exchange Commission to sell stocks, bonds, mutual funds, and a broad range of other investments. Ideally, a good broker acts as a long-range adviser; that is, he or she will tailor the components of a portfolio to your expressed investment goals by consulting with you, keeping you informed of new opportunities, and helping you determine what and when to buy and what and when to sell. In reality, however, it doesn't always work that way, especially for the small investor. Brokers make commissions on every transaction they make for you, so you'd better be prepared to make the decisions and monitor the activity.

Tax Preparation Services: The best known is H & R Block, but there are others, including independent individuals, who prepare taxes. The IRS also offers assistance. If you've kept good records and your taxes are relatively simple, then using one of these services is fine. In fact, the IRS hotline or one of their publications may be all you need to complete your taxes yourself. Regardless of who prepares your taxes, however, even if it's a CPA, *you,* not the preparer, will be held accountable and responsible if you are audited and there are errors in your returns. (See more about income taxes in the next chapter.)

Consumer Credit Counseling Service: Mainly used for debt consolidation and reduction strategies. Discussed earlier, see pages 154–155.

Insurance Agents and Underwriters: These are the first financial advisors you're likely to develop a relationship with, and some say the most important. (See the next chapter for a more complete discussion of insurance coverage.)

Director of Employee Benefits: Here is an advisor whose services are free, but who is generally overlooked simply because he or she is sitting right in your company down in the personnel/human resources department. Sadly, most employees have little knowledge, much less any understanding, of their total employee benefits package. Through where you work, you may already have, or be able to obtain, health and life insurance, disability protection, retirement and pensions funds, profit sharing, and additional investment opportunities. How can you know what you need if you don't know what you have? Check it out—today!

What Next?

So far, we've been talking about monitoring cash flow and using credit, the day-to-day strategies for staying solvent. Solvency is a first step to any kind of financial stability, of course, but you want more than that. You want to get ahead. For that, you'll have to be a little more forward thinking and put some long-term strategies in place. And for advice on how to do that, you'll have to go on to Chapter 9.

CHAPTER 9

Building Financial Security: Long-Term Goals

Nobody needs to tell newlyweds that life is uncertain. Accidents happen, companies fold, investments fail, new obligations arise, and nobody means to imply that financial security alone will protect against every mishap and heartbreak. But if couples don't do better than just living paycheck to paycheck, and if they don't develop the skill and discipline needed to build a solid financial foundation, then they remain vulnerable to the adverse effects of every changing circumstance that can conceivably come along.

This chapter takes the long view: planning for major purchases, such as a home, and protecting yourselves against unexpected misfortune, such as illness or unemployment. Besides accumulating property and protecting assets, it's also nice if you can build some wealth and security for your "golden years." To that end, we will discuss insurance, debt reduction, savings and investments, and income tax planning. We'll even show you how a certified financial planner devised a long-term plan for a typical newlywed couple.

If there's one message that's emerged from all the financial upheaval of the last few decades, it's that couples are going to have to take charge of their own affairs and plan for their own future security. They cannot depend on their relatives, employers, or government in the same way that previous generations might have. Along with challenge comes opportunity, however. Regardless of the prevailing economic climate, there will always be those who turn the situation to advantage, maintain the perseverance to achieve their dreams, even manage to accumulate great wealth.

Whatever your goals are, you can attain them because you two are a couple now. You have twice the talent, twice the potential, and twice the resources at your disposal. You can use that double strength to redouble your determination, not only to survive, but to succeed.

❧ *Do You See Yourself Here?* ❧

- Are you confused about where to begin to identify your long-term financial goals?
- Do you have trouble prioritizing those goals or agreeing on how to reach them?
- Has either of you brought a negative financial history to this partnership?
- Do you feel vulnerable to disaster: the loss of a job, a sudden illness, an unexpected financial obligation?
- Are you as a couple dealing with the effects of one of these disasters right now?
- Do you feel totally out of your league discussing taxes, insurance, investments, and other wealth-building, wealth-protecting topics?
- Are you hoping to buy a house, return to school, or make some other large financial investment soon?
- Do you fear the IRS?

Yes? Keep reading.

Setting Goals

Norma and Calvin come from remarkably similar socioeconomic backgrounds: both were raised by single mothers who struggled to make ends meet, both started working and handling their own money in high school, and both put themselves through college with a combination of jobs, loans, and scholarships. On the surface, at least, the couple would seem to be predictably alike in the way they think about money, yet that has turned out not to be the case at all.

"I just want to be able to live comfortably without worrying about finances all the time," says Norma. "To me, that would be luxury enough, but not to Calvin. He's shooting for real luxury, real wealth, complete financial independence so he can retire by the time he's 50. And all I want is a house."

The point: even the same backgrounds and the same experiences don't necessarily generate the same goals. And, even if you can agree on the same day-to-day methods of managing your budget, as Norma and Calvin easily have, you can still harbor very different ideas of where you want that day-to-day management to lead you.

This couple, at least, has admitted their different goals and thus set the stage for negotiating them. But they will have to compromise so that they can both agree on their priorities; otherwise, only one of them will be committed to the long-term task of building wealth. Without a unified commitment of both partners, achieving any financial goal is doubtful.

There are all kinds of goals, both intermediate and long-term, and nobody but you can decide what yours should be. Some couples just want to stay out of debt and build a comfortable cushion of financial reserves so they can stop worrying about every negative economic forecast; others want a house, or a college degree, or the freedom to stay at home while raising children. Others want still more—a vacation home, a luxury car, an impressive portfolio of stocks and bonds, a college education for children they haven't even had yet.

In short, there are as many kinds of goals and dreams as there are lifestyles and couples to live them. Before you begin any long-term financial planning, you have to determine what yours are.

Financial Planning Priorities

While experts can't tell you what your exact goals should be, virtually every expert consulted for these financial chapters agreed on the priority different types of goals should receive: that is, which *kinds* of goals are basic and should be taken care of first, which are intermediate and get accomplished along the way, and which are long-term and depend on a family's ultimate definitions of success and security.

Goals are always evaluated in terms of the monetary cost and the estimated time you think it will take you to reach them. Cost and time, of course, are affected by factors such as your age, income, risk tolerance, financial obligations, tax situation, and spending priorities. As with most things in life, one choice usually precludes another. Unless they're already wealthy, for instance, most couples are not going to be able to afford a luxury vacation every year while they're also trying to save for a house.

Financial planners are quick to point out that reaching longer-term goals usually requires short-term sacrifice. When people are not willing to defer instant gratification for future satisfaction, one of two things happens: either the goal is never reached, or enormous debt is incurred to have it all, now.

Following is a priority list for the various kinds of goals you might have. The rest of the chapter discusses each of them in more detail.

Planning Priorities

1. Safeguard what you have through adequate protection and emergency reserves.
2. Reduce debt and practice the judicious use of credit.
3. Save for intermediate goals: home, children, etc.
4. Establish financial security through building assets and making your money grow.
5. Achieve financial independence: retirement.

First Things First (Priority #1)

"At any age or any stage or any income level, nobody likes to hear this," says Agnes A. Roach, Certified Financial Planner and president of AA Roach Financial Planning, "but the absolute first priority for any couple or individual hoping to build any kind of financial security at all is to establish an emergency fund, a cash reserve to cover from three to six months' worth of expenses. I don't know of any financial planner anywhere who wouldn't strongly recommend this liquid fund as a basic necessity."

Using our average *Modern Bride* couple's income of $54,200, that means a fund of between $13,000 and $27,000 in the bank, just in case of emergency. This is not a fund to be used as an investment, because it must be kept liquid and readily available, and not a fund to be used toward an eventual purchase, such as a house or a car. It is simply a fund to be there, as protection, in case of the loss of a job or some other unexpected disaster.

It can take couples years to save it, and it's a lot of money to have just lying around in a bank account or credit union, especially when interest rates on savings are low. It's also awfully tempting to spend it once you've got it. No wonder so many people balk at this advice.

"I know, I know," Roach agrees, "it's hard to save that money and leave it alone. But speaking as someone who has seen clients unexpectedly lose their jobs, I know how important the security of such a fund can be, particularly in this economy."

If both of you are working, Roach advises, then you can probably get away with a three-month income reserve, but if one of you is not employed full-time, or if you both work for the same company, then you'd better plan for a six-month reserve. "Unemployment is devastating for anybody, but it can be particularly hard on a young person because there's usually not much severance pay offered, if any," says Roach. "And unemployment compensation doesn't begin to cover most people's living expenses, much less the costs of looking for another job."

Beyond the threat of unemployment, remember too that this is an overall emergency fund. You would turn to it not only in the case of job loss, but also for other needs, such as illness, repairs, unexpected family obligations, or insurance deductibles.

Insurance Protections

"Our entire financial situation has been determined by one single event early in our marriage," says Bonnie. "We will be getting out from under the cost of Ray's cancer for years to come."

This is the couple you met in Chapter 2 who faced the husband's treatment for testicular cancer eight months into their marriage. But four years later, with a new baby, Bonnie and Ray are still trying to reduce thousands of dollars' worth of medical debt through regular, systematic payments. The burden of this debt has recently forced them to rent out their own home in order to defray the monthly mortgage, and to move into a grandparent's house.

"When it comes to health, money is no object for someone you love," Bonnie says. "But we did learn a hard lesson through this, and we will never again make the same mistake." The mistake she refers to is not knowing the limitations of Ray's health insurance at work and not realizing, until they got into the situation, just how limited that coverage was and how vulnerable they were financially.

Most people are either overinsured or underinsured, and it takes savvy consumers to put together an adequate insurance package of health, life, disability, homeowners, and auto to cover every need and contingency. Don't let what you don't know hurt you. Study the insurance coverage you have from your employer and make an appointment with the appropriate benefits advisor to clarify anything you don't understand. Then, get recommendations from friends and relatives for reputable agents who can help you evaluate and determine any additional insurance needs (see Appendix for resources).

An Insurance Primer

Health Insurance: Of all the areas of financial vulnerability, healthcare costs lead the way. This is also the area most likely to change with ever-expanding government policies and national reforms. Until everyone is guaranteed protection against astronomical costs, however, it's up to you to establish your own safeguards.

Most people have health insurance through their employers. If you are both employed, you will need to carefully review both your policies to understand what they cover and to determine any duplication of benefits. Don't be too quick to reduce coverage or to relinquish a plan to which you must contribute, however, just because one of you has what seems like an adequate plan. Check the fine print, particularly the deductibles, maximums, and range of services covered.

Typical health plans cover in-hospital expenses, nursing care and supplies, surgical costs separate from hospital expenses, and major medical, which takes over where the other coverage leaves off. In addition, some policies also include dental care, eye exams, mental health professionals and family therapy, and other procedures and practices.

Sometimes, including your spouse on your plan means an additional cost to you. It may or may not be worth it. If one of you is not employed, of course, then the additional fee for the spouse, called a family plan, is advisable.

Today, with spiraling insurance costs, most companies are attempting to save by either reducing benefits or asking their employees to contribute. It goes without saying that any coverage you get for nothing should be maintained, and anything for which you contribute only a nominal fee should be given serious consideration.

Independent health insurance is, proportionately speaking, very expensive. If you are self-employed, look to industry associations and professional organizations for group plans that might be available to you as a member. You might also investigate health maintenance organizations (HMOs) as an economic alternative. (Some employers now offer HMOs as an alternative, too.)

Disability Insurance: This is protection against income loss due to an inability to work. Insurance companies define disability in different ways and have different qualifying standards and periods for releasing benefits. They also define their plans as two kinds: short-term, which have a shorter waiting period before benefits commence, but a finite pay-out period; and long-term, which are designed to address catastrophic circumstances.

Paid income benefits are a percentage of your salary, usually 60 to 80 percent, for a period of years or up to a certain age, depending on the type of coverage. You cannot collect disability benefits from two overlapping policies, but you can structure your coverage protection to compensate for the deficiencies of one plan with the benefits of another.

Most employers offer some sort of disability coverage as part of their standard benefits package. Find out. If you pay Social Security taxes, you are also entitled to protection under Social Security. If you are injured on the job, you are also eligible for protection under the Worker's Compensation laws. Check with your employer to find out more about that coverage in your state.

Life Insurance: The selection of life insurance is complicated by a broad range of plans available, and by a changing list of personal requirements that vary with your age, your income, and your family's financial needs. There are two basic kinds of life insurance: term, which gives the maximum death benefit with the lowest premium, but with no accrual of monetary value (some term insurance is "convertible," which means you can convert it to whole life later on); and whole life, which offers savings plus protection at a higher premium. There is also a range of products going by several names—universal life, endowment life, or variable life—that offer death benefits plus investment opportunities, along with a flexible payment schedule. You will have to educate yourself about these opportunities to see if any of them make sense for you.

In general, young couples with no children, little property, and few financial obligations should choose term insurance because it offers the most coverage for the least cost. If you have children or property, however, you will need more sophisticated coverage. Both of you should be covered by life insurance, even if one of you is not employed. Frankly, funeral costs alone would indicate the need for some coverage.

Again, if you are employed, chances are you already have some life insurance through work. Check to see what you have and find out how your plan can be adapted to meet new needs. And don't forget to add your spouse's name as beneficiary.

Homeowner's Insurance: Whether you own or rent, you will need homeowner's insurance. *Renters are not covered by their landlords' policies.* In terms of value, homeowner's insurance is the most inexpensive protection you can buy. Moreover, when you think about the cumulative worth of all your wordly possessions—furniture, appliances, stereo, wedding presents, etc.—you will agree that homeowner's insurance is not a luxury, but a necessity.

Homeowner's insurance fulfills two basic needs: 1. it protects the physical contents of your home against fire, theft, and other accidents; and 2. it offers liability coverage to protect current or future assets. Contents coverage helps you replace the contents of your home should they be lost, stolen, damaged, or vandalized. It covers the dwelling (if you own it) and everything in it.

Liability coverage protects you against damages should someone be injured on your property or should you somehow be responsible for accidental or bodily injury to someone somewhere else. Be sure to carry enough liability insurance to safeguard all your assets that could be at risk in a lawsuit. (Most home insurers offer an umbrella policy, for an additional $200 to $300 a year, that protects your home, your car, your business, and other assets up to $1 million in damage suits.)

To determine how much insurance you need, the National Association of Professional Insurance Agents recommends that you make a complete inventory of all your possessions, including taking photographs and listing estimated replacement values. (Inventory guides are available from many insurance companies and agents.) Once you have an inventory, then shop around for the best total plan for you.

Rates vary with types of coverage, and you may even need additional protection, called "insurance riders" or "personal property floaters," to cover special expensive items such as jewelry, furs, collections, antiques, etc. Also, if you live in an area where damage from floods, hurricanes, earthquakes, or other "Acts of God" is likely, you might want to investigate separate coverage for those circumstances, which are not usually included in a routine homeowner's policy.

Auto Insurance: Everyone who owns an automobile should have auto insurance, and most states require it. Auto insurance provides two types of coverage: collision, which protects you against the damage you do to your own car; and liability, which protects you against the losses you cause others by your carelessness.

Auto insurance costs are influenced by several factors, not the least of which are where you live and what kind of vehicle you drive. Your driving record, your age, sex, and marital status also affect your insurance rates (newlywed men will find that they finally get a break on insurance because of being married). Higher deductibles (the amount you pay before the insurance kicks in) will significantly reduce rates. If you elect all the various types of coverage offered, everything from towing to rental car fees to comprehensive coverage against winds and floods, you'll increase your premiums significantly.

It really pays to shop around for auto insurance, and to reevaluate your coverage and carrier from time to time. Often, if you do a "package deal," that is, purchase auto and homeowner's from the same insurer, you will get a price break. And, marriage often lowers rates for younger men. Check to see. If you can afford higher deductibles on any of your policies, you'll be able to reduce your premiums that way, too.

Reducing and Controlling Debt (Priority #2)

Mannie came to marriage with two maxed-out credit cards, for a total of $8,000, a four-year remaining car loan, to the tune of $479 a month, and department store charges that added up to just over $2,000. "To be perfectly honest," she says, "the wedding put us over the edge." She refers to the $1,800 wedding gown, which she charged, and the $6,000 honeymoon, which her husband charged. In short, the couple started out over with over $30,000 in consumer debt, and they hadn't even bought anything for their new life together yet!

"This is the kind of situation that causes me to amend my own advice about the emergency fund," says our financial planning expert, Agnes Roach. "Because for a couple with this much consumer debt at relatively high interest rates, accumulating savings, or an emergency fund, at much lower interest rates gets them nowhere fast. For them, I would recommend trying to address both savings and debt reduction at the same time. After basic expenses, they need to use half their discretionary monies to pay off the debt, and save the other half. It will take them twice as long to get to square one, but they have to get there before they can do anything else."

One of the rules of thumb everybody uses is that if you are paying more than 20 percent of your net income each month on consumer debt (excluding mortgage), you're in dangerous territory. Mannie and her husband had long since passed that earmark, so the debt had to be reduced before they could possibly hope to begin establishing any financial security, much less saving toward the accumulation of real assets.

Let's understand, though, that all debt isn't bad. Some, in fact, is necessary to build the kind of credit history that will allow you to undertake a debt that is worthwhile, such as a home mortgage. But experts agree that the purpose of establishing credit is to be able to borrow money for solid investment opportunities, not for everyday frills.

Shortfalls in the Short-Term

Financial experts make clear distinctions among the many types of debt; those that are assumed in the accumulation of real property—houses, investments, education, even cars—make more sense than those that are incurred for fleeting pleasures. Clothes, vacations, dinners out, and the like may be good for the psyche, but they do not generate real-world assets. Therefore, they do not constitute good uses of credit.

We already talked about controlling spending habits as a way to keep the monthly budget in line, but it becomes more than that. Each immediate choice translates into long-term priorities. Is driving/leasing an expensive sports car really worth postponing the purchase of your own home? Each time you get ready to make a short-term debt commitment, you need to evaluate that decision with a long-term perspective. Reducing and controlling debt is a close second in the priority list of achieving long-term financial goals. In some situations, it goes hand in hand with number 1, because you can't effectively safeguard what you have if you are vulnerable to a collection agency. Look for ways to consolidate debt and get it paid off so that you can keep it to controllable levels in the future. And don't be shy about getting the help you need through debt counseling to do it. Your future solvency, after all, depends on it.

About Your Credit Records

If you had department store charge cards, a bank card, or a car loan or lease before you were married, then you came to marriage with some sort of credit history. That history stays with you in marriage, so that if one of you had trouble paying bills on time, it is likely that you'll both suffer for that record.

With over 2,000 credit bureaus around the country, one or two of them will be located in your community and will have a file on you. You have a right to inspect that, and you should, especially if you find you are being consistently turned down for credit. Errors do happen, and an examination of your records affords you the opportunity to correct a negative report, or at least to file a letter of explanation. The Fair Credit Reporting Act requires credit bureaus to make your records available to you upon request, although they will charge a small fee. Look in the Yellow Pages under "credit reporting agencies" to find the numbers for those in your area.

Whenever you apply for credit, the local credit reporting agencies are consulted. Then, the loan application is evaluated on what is known as "the three Cs": character, which is your credit history and apparent trustworthiness; capacity, meaning your income and your presumed ability to pay; and capital, which is the collateral that exists to secure the loan (some loans, like bank credit cards, are unsecured). If you score well on these points, a lender is likely to approve the loan you seek; if not, you can try another lender, because standards often vary from one institution to another.

If you are turned down for a loan, you have the right, under the Equal Credit Opportunity Act, to know why. This act also prohibits lenders from discriminating on the basis of race, gender, or marital status. A man or a woman

---

What Other Couples Say . . .

Cars, vacations, kids—there are all kinds of dreams, but owning your own home is still number 1 for today's couples, just as it has been for generations. Fifty-three percent of the couples surveyed in a *Modern Bride* Consumer Council Study of Newlyweds (Cahners, July 1993) reported that they reside in a house or condo they own.

can apply for, and receive, credit in his or her own name, and you should do that. As we discussed in Chapter 8, both of you should have established credit as individuals and as a couple.

Saving to Make the Dreams Come True (Priority #3)

Lots of us don't save at all. Those who do, according to financial experts, save about 4 percent of their income on average. Yet, every expert recommends saving 10 percent of your income as a minimum, 15 to 20 percent if you're serious. Notice some disparity here...?

Newlyweds, particularly, feel "damned if they do, and damned if they don't." From one of them about saving for a house: "It's so frustrating. We've scrimped and saved and scrimped and saved and yet, when we go out looking, we still can't afford anything decent." From another about trying to get started: "How can we save? We just got out of school. We have to have dependable cars, clothes for work, some furniture for the apartment, appliances—all that stuff."

Frustration, postponement, other priorities—valid excuses all, but excuses that will impede the attainment of future dreams. You have to begin, and you have to begin today. Otherwise, you will *never* buy that house, own that car, get that degree, start that business, make that investment, or whatever else you might be striving toward.

We said in the last chapter that marriage, as a financial partnership, is supposed to make a profit. Saving is how you do it. Through savings, you have the money to achieve your dreams, to make more money, to fund investments, and to build assets. You will never reach financial security, much less any degree of wealth, if you just earn and spend, even if you don't spend more than you make.

Recently, the *Wall Street Journal* (August 6, 1993, B1) reported on a shocking study that found that over a third of all U.S. households have *no* discretionary income! That means that these families have no monies left over after meeting their basic expenses of food, clothing, housing, and taxes. How do they make it? How do they ever get ahead? The answer is, they don't.

Easing the Pain of Sacrifice

Saving is never easy, but there are ways to make it less painful. Consider these strategies:

- Set a savings goal and stick to it. Back to our average *Modern Bride* couple with an income of $54,200: a 10 percent savings rate on after-tax income would mean socking aside roughly $4,000 a year, or about $333 a month. But in ten years, at a compounded growth rate of just 5 percent, they would have almost $60,000. Think of it this way: the years are going to pass anyway. What are you going to have to show for them?

- Pay yourselves first. Even if it's as little as $50 or $100 a pay period, it's something. Saving less sooner in life builds more, over the long haul, than saving more starting later. For example, if one saves just $100 a month starting at age 30, and it grows tax free at roughly 10 percent a year to age 65, it will grow to $379,272 in those 35 years. But, if one doesn't start to save until age 40, that same $100 a month will only grow to $132,593 in 25 years. It pays to start early!

- If you both work, live on one and one-half salaries. Make that a lifelong practice. Not only will you start to build wealth, but you'll be able to fund extraordinary expenses, such as putting a kid through college, without extraordinary sacrifice in your lifestyle.

- Take advantage of pretax savings and investment plans through where you work. (In some companies, employers will contribute to your funds, which means someone else is helping you save!) At first, you'll miss the monies deducted automatically from your paycheck, but you'll learn to live on less.

- Ditto with automatic transfers from your checking account to a savings account or money fund at your bank.

- Shop around for the best investment vehicles for your money. Remember: **these savings are in addition to your emergency fund,** so they don't have to remain liquid. The idea here is to make money, even when interest rates are low. Look for mutual funds that rely on diversified investments, and plan to leave your money invested long enough (usually about three years) to realize some gains.

- Don't adjust your lifestyle upward with every pay raise or apparent windfall. There will be times, of course, when your standard living expenses will have to increase (when buying a house or having a family, for instance), but for most people, increased taxes, additional contributions to employee healthcare, and flat rates of return on investments will continue to put the squeeze on the amount of take-home pay, even if salaries go up. "Nobody will be sorry if they adopt the conservative approach to living in this economic climate," says Roach.

Buying a Home

Buying a home is a hot topic among newlyweds, probably because home ownership is still the cornerstone of the American Dream as far as most people are concerned. On the practical side, owning a home has many advantages. For about the same as you pay in rent (maybe for less in periods of low interest rates), you can carry a home mortgage and build equity. You can enjoy the pride and pleasure of ownership, plus have tax deductions because of it. And, in a good real estate market, you can parlay your present house into a bigger, better one, thereby realizing a significant return on a capital investment.

But, there is a downside, too, one that first-time homeowners often forget at their peril. The downside is that you *do* own it, complete with all the repairs, maintenance, taxes, problems, and other liabilities that come along. When something goes wrong, you can't call the super; you are the super, and wells and water heaters and septic tanks and driveways and decks and dishwashers and roofs and rafters can all give you a super headache, too. But, hey, that's part of the dream, isn't it?

Your decision to buy a home will depend on what's available in the market, how favorable interest rates are, and how financially prepared you are to make the initial purchase and to sustain the ongoing responsibility. You also have to be honest with each other about your lifestyle priorities, and your willingness to sacrifice to own a home. Making the leap to home ownership is a big step, one that will put additional demands on your time, money, and patience. Only you can determine when the move is right, but here are some things you should think about as you start looking.

Purchase price: Different groups recommend different guidelines, from two to three times your annual income is usual. The American Bar Association recommends two and one-half times, which sounds reasonable. That means our *Modern Bride* couple with an income of $54,200 would be looking at a house costing no more than about $135,000. Obviously, if you have a great deal of money to put down, that would adjust this guideline upward.

Down payment: The standard is 20 percent of the purchase price, but some lenders will accept 10 percent. The greater your down payment, the lower your total mortgage, so the lower your monthly payment will be, depending on interest rates. However, when figuring the down payment, don't forget about the closing costs (fees for appraisal, survey, title search, attorney, taxes in escrow, lender's points, etc.) you'll have to pay when you actually sign the contract. In some areas, these costs can run into thousands of dollars.

Further, don't forget the monies you'll need or want right away when you move in to make the place livable. This is particularly true if you're purchasing "a handyman's special" that needs lots of work. You don't want to strap yourselves so tightly that you won't be able to enjoy some of the fun of fixing up.

Monthly mortgage payments: How much can you afford? Again, there are all sorts of guidelines, the most common one being the one set by Fannie Mae (The Federal National Mortgage Corporation) some years ago: total housing expense (including mortgage, property taxes, homeowner's insurance, and any other fees and assessments) should not exceed 28 percent of your gross income. Most financial advisers think that's pretty high, especially if a couple has other debt, such as car loans, student loans, etc.

Ultimately, you have to decide what you can afford, and sometimes you have to decide fast when interest rates are moving, because the interest rate at which you secure your mortgage, and the kind of mortgage you secure, make big differences in the monthly payments. Basically, you can estimate that each percentage point in interest equals about $75 a month on a $100,000 mortgage. On a 30-year, fixed-rate $100,000 mortgage, that would look like this:

6%	7%	8%	9%	10%	11%	12%	13%	14%	15%
$600	$665	$733	$804	$877	$952	$1,028	$1,106	$1,184	$1,264

Remember, now, this does *not* include taxes, insurance, or any other maintenance costs.

Mortgage types: There are many way to finance a home, and each has certain advantages for certain types of couples and incomes. The most common mortgage types are: the **fixed-rate mortgage,** for 15, 25, or 30 years, which means a "fixed" interest rate and equal monthly payments spread out over the life of the loan; **variable-rate** or **adjustable mortgage,** which allows interest rates, and therefore the monthly payment, to fluctuate over the life of the loan; and **graduated payment** and **balloon mortgages,** both forms of a buy-now-pay-later method that assumes a higher income and, consequently, a greater ability to pay in the future.

Shop around on this, for both competitive interest rates and mortgage types. But mortgage agreements can be very complicated, so be sure you understand what you're getting into before you sign.

Stability and Security (Priority #4)

You might get some variation on the theme of financial security, but basically, the term means achieving a level of stability that isn't threatened by every unexpected turn of events. In other words, if one of you loses a job, or the market takes a swift downturn, or you need a new roof on the house, the two of you will be able to withstand the temporary setback without ending up in bankruptcy court. We're not talking complete financial independence here, and certainly not independent wealth, but a level of security that allows you to sleep at night.

Stability—a worthy goal in an unstable world, and a goal that can be achieved, although perhaps not right away. The other things we've already talked about have to be in place first: a regular savings and investment plan; protection for life, health, and property; a solid credit rating; an absence of inordinate debt; and the early acquisition of assets that will grow in value. Given steady employment and wise money management, this kind of financial security can be yours in just a few years. And from there, you can go on to pay for kids' college educations and live comfortably in retirement, even build real wealth if that is your dream.

Nobody says this is easy, especially in a "want it all now" world where the pressures to buy, consume, and enjoy are unrelenting. Unexpected expenses will crop up, and momentary desires will overwhelm, and then you will have to reevaluate, readjust, maybe even re-resolve and start again.

On top of human weakness, you also have to separate the romance of your dreams from the reality of your earnings potential:

- How stable is the industry in which you work?
- What are your chances of increasing your income/position over the years?
- Should you address educational needs in order to improve your earnings potential?
- What secondary sources of income might you be able to develop through talents, interests, hobbies, or skills?

Besides common sense, couple communication, and good money management, a big part of successful financial planning depends on the realistic appraisal of your goals in light of your resources. (Winning the lottery, for instance, is not a realistic expectation.) Being brutally honest in that appraisal now, as newlyweds, works to great advantage because you are in a position to change your potential, through changing careers, or going back to school, or relocating to another area of the country. As you get older, and more entrenched in your lifestyle habits, these changes are harder to make, but the regrets from not having made them will come all too easily.

Independence and Wealth (Priority #5)

To most people, the point of working and saving their whole lives is so they can live comfortably, and independently, in their later years. Obviously, definitions of wealth, even of comfort and independence, vary and may change over the years.

Although you may already be contributing to pension funds and profit sharing where you work, most newlyweds are too busy trying to figure out how to get started financially to worry about how they will end. So, we won't dwell on this topic.

However, there are two things you should think about now: 1. tax-deductible, tax-deferred retirement programs (such as IRAs, Keogh plans, 401K plans, annuities, and others) offer tremendous opportunities to build wealth while reducing present tax liability; and 2. the wealth you build, particularly in salary-deferred plans, is a form of savings that does not necessarily have to be used for retirement. Often, you can borrow against these funds, or even withdraw them (although you will pay a penalty for early withdrawal). If automatic deductions are being made out of your paycheck, make sure that you know exactly what they are for, and that you can take with you whatever *you* have contributed to an employee retirement plan should you leave that employment. If you have not worked there long enough to be "vested," you could lose a substantial amount. Find out how long it takes to be vested, and what happens if you leave before you are.

The Tax Collector Cometh

You'd better believe it! He cometh once a year, on April 15, for regular working people, and he cometh four times a year, every quarter, for the self-employed. Miss a date with him, and you'll wish you were dead, which is the only other certainty in life besides the tax collector.

The IRS is an awesome institution and its operating procedures are contained in several thousand pages of tax codes stipulating rules and regulations that are constantly changing. The mere mention of a tax audit is enough to send a stalwart heart into arrythmia, and arguments over what's right and what's wrong, what's allowed and what's disallowed, drag through the tax courts for years. Indeed, even advisors on the other end of the IRS tax hot line give conflicting advice! How then can you hope to emerge sane and solvent from this quagmire of deductions and exemptions?

There is only one answer that will save you—save you money, save you aggravation, and save you should you ever be audited—and that answer is "records." You must keep adequate records, at least of everything you earn and everything you make, and also of anything you spend that might be an allowable deduction. The more complicated your financial affairs, the more records you'll have to keep, but you can keep them anywhere: in a shoebox, in a file cabinet, or in a computer's memory. And, by the way, you should keep those records for three years after the filing year.

Whether you prepare your income taxes or you have a professional do it, the efficiency and the success of the task will depend on the accuracy of the records you keep. A lawyer or tax accountant is not about to declare anything that he or she can't prove, and neither should you. Tax fraud means heavy fines and penalties, even jail, and ignorance is no excuse.

On the other hand, nobody, not even Uncle Sam, expects you to pay more in taxes than you are legally required to, so figuring taxes and deductions accurately is in your own best interest. Yes, you'll eventually get a refund check if you overpay during the course of the year, but why let the government use your money interest free? Why not have the use of it all year long yourselves? And yes, if you underdeduct during the year, you'll have to cough up what you owe when you file, and that can be a real blow to the budget!

Romantic Returns

Most people don't associate romance with the IRS, but Hector and Cathy do. She explains why:

"Once a year, usually at the end of January, we declare a tax-preparation weekend. We make no other plans, allow no interruptions, and literally shut ourselves up together for two whole days. We gather all our records and purchase a good tax-preparation guide before the weekend, and I plan in advance for two lovely, easy, romantic dinners.

"Then we go at it. We work all day and relax in the evenings. If it turns out we owe, we hold our return until April 15; if we're due a refund, we congratulate ourselves, and send in the return early. Either way, we've had a nice, quiet, productive winter weekend together."

Just goes to show that romance can be found wherever you look for it!

There is a bigger message to Cathy and Hector's story, however, and that is that tax law is complicated and ever changing. Unless you keep good records all year long, and unless you are willing to make a concerted effort in studying up to fill out your own returns, you may be better off using the help of a professional. It can cost quite a bit to have them professionally prepared if your tax returns are complicated and involve many forms. Be sure you know what the fees are before you enlist the aid of a professional preparer, and find out if those fees include any tax advice for the next year. Also, should you get audited, will this tax preparer represent you before the IRS (generally, only lawyers or CPAs can represent you), or at least accompany you?

If you decide to tackle your taxes yourselves, there are excellent computer software programs available for tax preparation, as well as new books published each year that explain the current tax laws, and the ramifications of any recent changes. Computer software is modestly priced, and reference books are not expensive at all. But it will take you some time to review these resources and learn how to use them, so they ought to be purchased well before the April 15 deadline.

How and When to File

Generally, among married couples, those filing jointly have the lowest tax rates, although you may want to do a preliminary run-through both ways, married filing singly and married filing jointly, to be sure. You may file a joint return as long as you were married during that filing year, even if the wedding was on December 31. Couples often complain that they feel penalized for being married, since single persons get higher deductions as individuals than married individuals do, but you *must* note your status as married and abide by the rules, and the different tax tables, that apply to married filers.

The completed tax forms, plus a check for whatever you owe, is due, postmarked, no later than midnight, April 15. You may file for an extension (for the paperwork, but not for an estimated tax payment), which gives you another three months, and you can even get extensions on your extensions. But the chore doesn't seem to get any easier with time.

The IRS provides basic filing information along with the 1040 form, and it also offers additional free booklets and information. Look for the 800 number to call, or the order blank for additional forms and specialized instruction booklets, in the back of your basic tax preparation guide. If you moved after you married, you may need to get new forms sent to your new address, or pick up blank forms. You can get forms and information from your public library as soon as they are made available from the IRS, generally in late January or early February.

Regardless of who fills out the forms, you both are responsible for the accuracy of your tax returns because both your names appear on the forms. If you are audited and found in error, you will both be held liable. If a couple files jointly, each is responsible for the entire tax debt. The IRS is not a tolerant taskmaster; when your bill is due, it's due. If you are late, interests and penalties mount up fast. That is why accurate record keeping and careful compilation are so very important.

Income Tax Checklist

Here are common records you as newlyweds might need to substantiate the various aspects of your tax return. Make it a habit to keep canceled checks and bank and investment statements, and collect records and receipts all year long to make your job at tax time easier.

- Wage and salary receipts—W2 forms
- Income from interest and dividends—statements
- Income from other sources—rent, royalties, tips, self-employment, inheritance, unemployment, gambling, etc.
- Capital gains income—from sale of real estate, personal property, stocks, etc.
- Losses—from investments, theft, casualty, gambling
- Home office expenses (mainly for self-employed)—percentage of rent/house payment, utilities, maintenance, equipment, insurance, etc.
- Deductions—mortgage interest and points, alimony, self-employment tax, self-employed health insurance and retirement plans, savings withdrawal penalties
- Taxes paid—federal, state, local, personal property, real estate, luxury, other
- Charitable donations—receipts for donations, mileage records for charity work
- Moving expenses—including the cost of looking for work
- Unreimbursed job-related expenses—union dues, auto, entertainment and travel receipts
- Dependent care—child, elderly, disabled
- Medical expenses—unreimbursed by insurance
- Tax preparation fees—cost of reference books, software, or professional fees

Note: This list is by no means exhaustive (although it may seem exhausting). Check actual IRS forms and schedules to see what other records you might need for your particular filing situation.

Creating a Long-Term Financial Plan

Where do you go from square one? We asked Agnes Roach, our consulting financial planner, to walk us through a long-term plan for our typical *Modern Bride* couple with an income of $54,200, just as she would if this couple came into her office. Here's what she advised.

Assuming that our couple has an emergency fund equal to at least three months' income and basic insurance covering health, disability, property, and life in place, the next consideration is how to invest the $333 monthly amount they can save. First, they need to list their financial objectives, deciding what they want to buy, how much each objective costs currently, and when they would like to attain it. Some typical objectives might look like this:

1. Establish a basic emergency fund equal to three months' income ($13,550 in this case) in a liquid account such as a bank or money market. (We're assuming this is in place.)
2. Carry basic health, disability, and life insurance protection—we're assuming this is all through the employer. Be sure there is adequate property insurance

on home, contents, and auto, complete with special riders for jewelry, art, etc. This, too, should be in place.

3. Take a tour of Europe in four years. Cost: $8,000 now.
4. Replace one automobile in six years. Cost now: $14,000.
5 Buy a home (or a larger home) in five years. Cost: $150,000. Need additional funds added to current equity or need a down payment of at least $15,000.
6. Save to start a family. Estimated cost: $1,000 for baby furniture, clothing, toys, etc. Time frame—three to four years.
7. Begin to contribute regularly to retirement accounts, mainly through participation in employer's plans.
8. Work with an attorney to draft a will. Cost: $300.

Once all objectives have been listed, it is necessary to prioritize them by importance. Since we're assuming numbers 1 and 2 are already in place, we'll look at numbers 3 through 8.

Since number 8 has the shortest time frame, the lowest cost, and possibly a large effect on this couple's future, we'll put that first. Number 7 will determine the couple's lifestyle in the future, so that becomes number 2. Let's assume that number 6 is next, followed by numbers 4, 5, and 3. These priorities are related strictly to the *couple's* order of importance. Now the list of objectives looks like this:

Objective	Cost	Time	Money Available
Draft wills	$300	now	A month's savings
Retirement (husband)	$100	now	Begin next month
Retirement (wife)	$100	now	Begin next month
Save for family	$1,000	3-4 yrs.	$133/mo. to invest
Auto	$14,000	6 yrs.	in a mutual fund
Home	$15,000	5 yrs.	for 4 to 6 years,
Tour Europe	$8,000	4 yrs.	starting next month

Realistically, based on current savings, not all these objectives can be achieved. However, if we assume an annual after-tax return of 7 percent in a growth and income mutual fund, then investing $133 a month for 5 years would yield up to $9,522, plus dividends and capital gains. This is not enough for all four goals, but it does yield enough for a healthy down payment on a car or part of the down payment on a house or a trip, depending on circumstances at the time.

Stating goals opens a path for a couple to follow, and it makes future choices easier. If one of you receives a raise, or if unexpected income from a gift or bonus is received, it is easier to decide what to do with it. It can be added to money saved toward stated goals. This will help avoid frivolous spending and ensure that mutually agreed upon priorities are followed.

CHAPTER 10

Understanding the Law

W alter proposed in one state, he and Sarah married in another, and now they live and work in a third. They are not unusual. From hometown, to college, to residency, many of the projected 2.5 million couples who marry each year will live under different jurisdictions and will make numerous legal and financial decisions during their lives together. And although today's brides and grooms are older and better educated than ever before, most have only a vague idea of what their marriage means legally, and how fundamentally important state and federal laws can be in the choices they make.

From the moment two people say "I do," their obligations to family and society, as well as to each other, begin to grow. Because society is a system of laws and values that allow us to live in harmony with one another, and because the family is the most basic unit of society, the government has a vested interest in the success of every union. In return, laws exist to ensure equity of rights and privileges, and to encourage marital stability.

Unfortunately, most people don't bother to find out what those laws are until difficulties arise—death, divorce, financial problems, or health catastrophes. But, by then, it is often too late to benefit from the protection the laws can afford, and newly discovered legalities can even make a bad situation more complicated.

Don't let the law take you by surprise. Now that you are an economic, as well as a social partnership, you need to find out all you can about the legal rights you have to help you protect and preserve your union. You also need to educate yourselves well enough to construct and implement your own legal safeguards where the letter of the law, as it exists, is lacking. The more you know about the legal ramifications of your decision to marry, the more secure your marriage will be, both financially and emotionally.

What Is Marriage?

There must have been times when it seemed like the whole world was going to be involved in your marriage. As you no doubt discovered during the months of wedding planning, marriage is not just a private act between two people; it's a public act in which family, community, and the state have a vested interest.

Do You See Yourself Here?

- Are you ignorant of the legal definition of marriage?
- Did you marry with a prenuptial agreement?
- Have you (the woman) decided to keep your maiden name, or to hyphenate your new name?
- Did either or both of you bring real property to the marriage?
- Are you totally unaware of the property laws that affect married couples in your state?
- Does either of you have assets that must remain separate property during the marriage?
- Have you moved to a state other than the one in which you were married or lived before marriage?
- Have you neglected to draw up a will?
- Are you without protection and contingencies should one of you become seriously ill or incapacitated?
- Are you (the woman) unsure of your reproductive rights under the law?
- Are you contemplating adoption?
- Has either of you been married before, with dependent children, receiving or paying alimony?
- Do the two of you own and operate a business together, or are you considering doing so?
- Have your circumstances (in terms of wealth, property, children, etc.) changed dramatically since the first year or two of marriage?

It is vitally important that you look into the issues involved in any "yes" answers. Read on for more.

Current trends toward cohabitation, delayed marriage, remarriage, divorce, lengthy litigations, and bitter custody battles have combined to create a new awareness of the seriousness of the marital contract, and the far-reaching consequences that contract, once made, can have on people's lives. Regardless of the flush of love and the romance of the honeymoon, it is important for all couples to understand the nature of the marriage contract into which they've entered.

Whereas most civil agreements can be easily changed, adapted, or even terminated by mutual consent of the parties involved, it is not so with marriage. Once this contract comes into existence, the legal status of the union may not be limited, altered, or dissolved without the consent of the state. Government is, in effect, an interested and participating third party.

The landmark decision in the U.S. Supreme Court case *Maynard v. Hill,* (1888) explains why: "It [marriage] is an institution in whose maintenance and purity the public is deeply interested. For it is the foundation of the family and society, without which there would be neither civilization nor progress." Those are pretty strong words.

As a social institution, then, marriage merges the assets and liabilities, and to some extent the identities, of two separate individuals into one functioning unit. By definition, this is supposed to be a profitable partnership. The government expects to share in that profitability through taxes, benefits, and allocations of resources. If the unit ceases to function properly, the government will step in to arbitrate and to protect its own interest in the welfare of the parties involved. As one newlywed put it at tax time, "Love may be between two people, but marriage is between two people and the state."

Obligations of the Contract

"I don't think most newlyweds fully appreciate the extent of the responsibilities you have for each other once you get married," says Bari, herself a newlywed and an attorney. "It doesn't really hit you until you start the business of married life—managing money, accruing property, planning for the future. Then one day you realize, oh my, I really am in partnership with this person, in every conceivable way!"

Asked to define marriage, most couples would probably describe it as a partnership. They would point to the fact that they both work, that they both share household responsibilities, and that they both care for family and children. There are, of course, couples who follow the more traditional divisions of labor in that partnership, and there are couples who totally reverse the traditional roles. In general, though, however the couple chooses to interpret their individual roles in the mutual support of each other in marriage is entirely up to them.

Marriage is a stable and convenient personal arrangement, a practical way to promote financial security, strengthen intimate family bonds, and raise children. Neither the state nor the society particularly cares who does what to effect this arrangement, as long as the partnership works.

The obligations you have to each other under the law are relatively few: each of you owes the other financial support; the two of you are expected, though not required, to live together; you are expected, and in some states required, to be sexually faithful; and neither of you must deny the other sexual intimacy without good cause. Although some obligations might be "enforceable" by law, in practical terms, if one partner consistently fails in these obligations, the only real recourse the other has is the dissolution of the marriage.

All states have, in some way, altered their laws to reflect changing times and to make gender-based roles in marriage obsolete. A man and a woman are expected to be mutually responsible for their own and their children's welfare. If one spouse is in need, for instance, the other must provide such basics as food and shelter, and that "other" may mean the wife, as well as the husband. The law attempts to be gender-blind; that's why, these days, the courts might require a wife to pay alimony, or award custody of the children to the father.

It is important to remember that marriage and family law is constantly changing to meet new needs and to reflect new societal attitudes. According to one family law practitioner, the changing status of women in society has done more to shape court decisions in marriage cases than any lawyer or judge ever could. The rising popularity of the premarital agreement is a good example of the ongoing evolution of family law.

Premarital Agreements

One legal tool that may supersede state statutes regarding marital property and inheritance rights is the premarital agreement drawn before the marriage. Also called a prenuptial or antenuptial agreement, this contract is designed to anticipate areas of possible dispute between people (and families), and to settle them in advance of the marriage. Typically, these agreements are most useful in prearranging financial matters and safeguarding inheritance rights, especially where children from a former marriage are involved.

If you have a premarital agreement, then you are probably aware of its clauses. Perhaps you incorporated automatic expiration dates or conditions for reevaluation into your agreement. Called "termination" or "sunset" clauses, these modifications not only recognize the inevitability of changing circumstances in a marriage, but also affirm a couple's belief that their marriage will last.

In order for the agreement to remain useful and valid, you should not intentionally violate any of its provisions. Of course, just as with the marriage contract itself, if any provisions are broken, one's only real recourse is the court, probably divorce court.

There is such a thing as a "postnuptial" agreement, entered into after the marriage, which is similar in form and content to a prenuptial, but usually entered into for different reasons. A postnuptial might be drawn when there has been a dramatic change in circumstances rather suddenly after the marriage, or when a couple is experiencing marital difficulties. Postnuptials are not as common as prenuptials, however, and their validity under your state's laws would have to be evaluated.

Changing Names

"The way I figure it, I've had this name for almost 31 years. Everyone, my family, my friends, and my colleagues, know me by it, so why should I change it because of some patriarchal custom?" says Serina, a newlywed who has steadfastly maintained her maiden name. "Ben says he understands, and I think he does, although I doubt he'd be as neutral in his feelings about our children's names."

In fact, Serina is right. The taking of a man's surname after marriage has always been just a custom, never a law, in the United States. An increasing number of women have reservations about honoring the custom, and an increasing number of men are bothered by their reluctance. So, what you have are hyphenated surnames, for both the wives and the husbands, or blended names, which are creative composites of both surnames, or a new last name altogether. Some couples even discuss which surnames the children will carry.

No state requires a name change. Generally, if you decide to assume a name, such as most women do after marriage, all you need to do is change it on your driver's license, credit cards, Social Security card, etc., and be consistent in its use. As long as a new name is not being assumed in order to defraud or escape prosecution, you are free to use whatever name you wish.

The problem, however, is that name changes have been used for fraudulent purposes, so much so that you will often now need proof, such as a marriage license, to show that you are who you say you are and that there is a legitimate reason for assuming a new name. Don't be surprised if you are questioned when you go to change the name on your passport, or your Social Security card, or your driver's license.

If you begin to use your husband's name after marriage, or you continue to use your own, there will be no problem as long as you're consistent. But, if your husband is going to change his, or if the two of you are going to settle on a new name, or if you change your mind at some point in the future, you are probably well advised to go to court to make the change official. (Often, a woman's maiden name is officially reestablished as part of a divorce proceeding.)

"It really is a question of identity," says Serina, "and I feel strongly about it. I know that traditionally many consider it proper to refer to me as Mrs. Ben —, but I don't even want to honor that tradition socially. Designation of marital status is no more important to a woman's identity than it is to a man's, and I don't want to perpetuate a sexist system."

Who Owns What?

Time was when the identity of a married couple, legal, financial, and otherwise, was based solely on the identity of one partner: the husband. But no more. The passage of the Married Women's Property Acts assured women the right to own property and to maintain their financial independence without their husband's control.

The increasing number of first marriages between working professionals in their late twenties and early thirties means that there are likely to be assets, and sometimes liabilities, brought to the marriage. The property that you bring to marriage is called **separate property,** and each of you can retain control over that property. Separate property includes such things as a car or boat, a condo or house, land, income-producing real estate, a business, artwork or collectibles, an inheritance or trust fund, stocks, bonds, or even jewelry. It may also include any inheritance or gifts given specifically to you during the marriage.

Separate property belongs to you, and may be bought, sold, or used as collateral for a loan, *as long as you keep it separate.* Be aware, however, that you relinquish sole ownership and control when you place an asset into a jointly held account or under a joint title. Once property loses its separate identity, your spouse, or creditors, may have legal claim to it. Also, if you use income from separate property to pay family expenses, it is generally considered an irretrievable "gift" to the family.

Ordinarily, couples don't worry about mingling their separate property, often because it doesn't even occur to them to think about it. But you might want to think about it, especially if you are in a position to be the beneficiary of a significant family inheritance, if you own and operate a business (alone or with other partners), or if you are financially responsible for a dependent family member. Check with an attorney, particularly if your property is sizable or your personal obligations great.

Laws of Ownership

Eight states are what are known as **community property** states: Arizona, California, Idaho, Louisiana, Nevada, New Mexico, Texas, and Washington, plus Puerto Rico. (Wisconsin follows the Uniform Marital Property Act, which makes it similar to a community property state.) Community property is a theory of ownership which assumes that whatever property is acquired by either partner after the marriage takes place, including wages, purchases, even pension funds, belongs to the community, that is, to both partners in the marriage. Besides meaning that all marital assets would probably be distributed evenly in the event of divorce, living in a community property state means that one spouse can be held responsible for the debts incurred by the other because all assets belong to both partners.

The other 41 states are known as **equitable distribution** states. Interestingly, equitable distribution is not a theory of ownership, but a concept by which property is distributed in the event of the dissolution of the union. In these states, there is no legal presumption that property acquired during the marriage belongs to both spouses. Rather, it is the way the property is held that determines ownership, and the way the court interprets fairness that determines distribution.

It is important for you to know what kind of state you live in because those laws guide how your property would be considered and distributed in the event of divorce or death. Effects can be far reaching, especially when you realize that college degrees and professional licenses acquired after the marriage are often considered property.

If either of you has significant separate property, or if the two of you have begun to accrue significant property together, you'll have to decide how you want to own things. Only by being familiar with your state laws can you make informed decisions regarding:

* How should the title to cars and the deed to houses be held?
* Can major property be disposed of without mutual consent?
* Should bank accounts and investments be in joint or separate names?
* What are your "rights of survivorship" in the event that one of you dies?

Whenever you move to another state during your marriage, be sure to have those decisions reevaluated in light of that new state's laws. See a local attorney, or call your state bar association for more information.

Who Owes What?

Just because you're married doesn't give either of you the right to saddle the other with monumental debts. Many states have what are called "family expense statutes," which make both spouses liable for debts incurred for the benefit of the family (groceries, child care, health care) even if one of them did not co-sign or approve of the expense. Except for these necessities, however, the theory of debt is pretty straightforward: if you bought it, you pay for it.

If you share an account with your spouse, you are both responsible of course. If you allow your spouse to use an account in your name, a credit card for instance, then you will be held accountable for all the charges on that account. If at any time you find you are unwilling, or unable, to pay the debts incurred by another in your name, then you must so notify the credit card company or individual merchant in writing.

Not very long ago, a woman didn't have to think about such things because she found it difficult to secure and maintain any credit in her own name. The Equal Credit Opportunity Act of 1974 changed all that. Now, discrimination due to race, color, age, religion, national origin, sex, or marital status when applying for credit is expressly prohibited.

While it is illegal to base the decision on a credit application solely on marital status, the fact is that creditors do treat married applicants differently than they do single ones. Sometimes, being married works to your advantage, as in a larger combined income or more personal stability. But, sometimes, differences in property rights, or a spouse's credit history, can work against you, too.

You should probably maintain some accounts and a credit rating in your name alone, in addition to your spouse's. That way, should something happen to your spouse, you won't have to reapply for existing loans and charge cards. You maintain an individual credit rating by using your own first name and surname (your new one if it changed after marriage). A woman should not use Mrs. John Doe, for instance, but Mrs. Mary Doe, on credit cards and bank accounts, even if those accounts are jointly held.

All businesses that offer charge accounts are required to keep account records in the names of both spouses, "if requested to do so." Request it. That way, even if one of you is a stay-at-home spouse or earns significantly less than the other, there will still be a personal credit history for each of you.

Inevitably, there is a certain blending of financial profiles between husband and wife, just as there is a blending of personal property, and that's fine because the two of you have to learn to work together and to trust each other. It's always wise, though, to be aware of your rights and your liabilities. (See more about credit and debt management in Chapters 8 and 9.)

Wills and Estates

"I just can't believe how John is acting about our wills," moans Nora, 32. "We have property, investments, and a child on the way, but he still persists in being childish himself. He ought to know better; after all, he's a lawyer!"

Regardless of his profession, John is suffering from an irrational fear of his own mortality—and he's not alone. Every year, thousands of people, people who should have known better, die "intestate" (without having made a will) and leave their families heir to monumental red tape, exorbitant legal fees, unnecessary taxes, and additional anxiety.

As soon as property starts to accumulate and children start to be born, wills should be drawn. If you die without one, your possessions, and your children, will be distributed according to the state's determination of kinship. While spouses are no doubt provided for in some way, the surviving spouse, especially when there are no children involved, may in fact be required to share the inheritance of property with the deceased's other living relatives.

In today's complicated legal climate, even couples who consider themselves of modest means might be surprised to find out what their estate is worth. (See the net worth exercise in Chapter 8.) Insurance, employee benefits, bonus programs, and other investments can make your estate worth considerably more than just the cars and a house. Couples need wills, as well as estate planning advice, to minimize tax liabilities for the survivors and to make sure assets are distributed as the deceased would wish.

Most attorneys would recommend drawing a will when a home is purchased, a child is born, or the net worth between you reaches a significant amount (about $100,000). Then again, the dollar amount doesn't really matter. If you want any control at all over how even modest possessions are distributed, then you should have a will. See an attorney to draw the will. Don't do it yourself! A simple one is not an expensive proposition; if your property is important enough to worry about, then it's important enough to consult someone to see that the legalities are properly handled.

Out-of-state wills and other previous agreements might be questioned in a new state. So, each time you move, it's a good idea to have an estate-planning

---

What Other Couples Say . . .

Far and away, the majority of newlywed couples interviewed, even newlyweds who are attorneys themselves, do not have wills. Most feel that either they don't have significant property or, in the case of those who are lawyers, they are comfortable with the intestate provisions of the state in which they live. (Couples who are not lawyers generally don't have a clue about property laws or intestate provisions in the state.) All say, however, that they would draw a will when a child is born, mainly because of the need to specify guardianship and to protect that child's inheritance.

conference and review existing documents with an attorney in your new state of residence.

Living Wills

The dramatic cases of extraordinary measures taken to preserve life have not only created several movies of the week on television, they have also created a new awareness, and even a fear, of the medical technology available to prolong life. The agonizing life-support decisions family members, and the courts, sometimes have to make have given rise to the increasing popularity of the living will and/or the durable power of attorney for health issues.

Perhaps you're aware of these legal tools for catastrophic illness because your parents or grandparents have enacted them. As Terry J. Barnett, an attorney, author, and authority on these documents, points out, "Medical technology exists today that can sustain life, even for years, in conditions that many people consider worse than death. Healthcare planning is not only for people who are old or sick. Accidents or unexpected illness can befall anyone."

A living will is a document, drafted and signed while you're able to make your own decisions, that expresses your wishes as to the extent of life-support systems and services you want to be employed in the event of your incapacity to make those choices for yourself. The durable power of attorney for health care is a document by which you transfer legal authority to make health and treatment decisions to someone else when you cannot make them for yourself. The power of attorney is not limited to life-sustaining procedures; it covers all healthcare decisions, unless you say otherwise in your document. It is "durable" because it empowers a person to make health decisions for you whenever you are mentally or physically impaired.

Terry Barnett favors the durable power of attorney because it vests the decision making in a real person. "Living wills are weaker planning instruments because no form can possibly anticipate every conceivable circumstance," he says. "Doctors and family members can feel very uncomfortable basing treatment decisions on a general expression of wishes."

If you have only a living will, your physician may ignore the document and defer to a family member, or the doctor may do whatever he or she would want for self or family members. A health care power of attorney tells your doctor that the representative you name is the person you want to make decisions for you and the person you want your doctor to talk with, just as the doctor would with you were you able to make your own decisions.

According to Barnett, you do not need an attorney to effect either a living will or a durable power of attorney, but you do need to be sure that the forms you use (available in stationery stores and most libraries, and in Barnett's book, see Appendix), are specific enough to offer direction. To be sure that they are helpful and do not conflict with state law, it wouldn't hurt to check your documents with an attorney who is experienced in medical matters.

People often say they don't want extraordinary means taken to preserve their lives when, in fact, they would if the odds in favor of full or partial recovery were in their favor. The real issue here is that you think about all of this very carefully, and be sure that you are enacting such provisions freely and with full understanding. Note, too, that if you decide to enact a durable power of attorney for health care, your spouse does not have to be named as your agent. Depending on your situation, a parent, a sibling, or a friend might be a better choice. Your goal is to choose the person you believe will be best able to represent your intentions regarding health care.

Reproductive Rights

Ideally, the decision to have a child is made mutually and belongs to the two of you. This right to privacy is guaranteed under the U.S. Constitution and it has been consistently upheld by federal and state courts. Except in the most extraordinary circumstances, the government plays no role in this decision, and neither does anyone else.

The law is concerned, however, with the rights and well-being of individual citizens, both adults and children. In 1965, *Griswold v. Connecticut,* the U. S. Supreme Court ruled that individuals have a right to obtain and use contraceptives if they do not wish to have a child. Subsequent cases have further established a woman's right to do what she likes with her own body.

That means you can use contraception, have a child, or have an abortion within the first trimester of pregnancy without the knowledge or consent of your husband. But, if either of you has concealed an unwillingness or an inability to have children from the other before marriage, that concealment may be grounds for divorce or annulment of the marriage. (As a matter of fact, any deliberate failure to disclose significant information before the marriage, such as a criminal record, an infectious disease, or sexual dysfunction, may be grounds for divorce or annulment.)

In the interest of public health and safety, the law also can determine where you have your baby, how it is delivered, and who attends the birth. State licensing boards and community regulations vary on home births and lay midwives, and the law gives doctors, and hospitals, considerable latitude in delivery room decisions. Your preferences and the options available should be discussed with your physician well in advance of pregnancy and birth.

You should also know that medically assisted pregnancies, through artificial insemination and in vitro fertilization, have varying legal implications in the different states. Make sure you know what these implications are if you are contemplating pregnancy by these means.

Once junior arrives, there are a multitude of children's rights laws to protect him, although many child advocates maintain that there still aren't enough. In general, you owe your children "reasonable support" according to your means, including maintenance and education, up to a certain age (usually 18 or 21).

You may use "reasonable force" to discipline your child, although some states have recently enacted laws to define and restrict that force.

The rights and responsibilities for adopted children are exactly the same as for natural children. All other issues related to child support and maintenance after divorce and the rights and responsibilities of stepparents who have not adopted their spouse's children are complicated and vary from state to state.

Marriage and family laws, particularly those that govern reproductive rights and the care and custody of children, are constantly changing to reflect changing roles, values, and even technology. Check with special-interest advocacy groups or your state bar association to find out more about specific laws that might affect your family life decisions.

Adoption

Adoption laws vary from state to state, and the legal system is very much involved in the adoption process. In all states, court approval is needed for the adoption to take place, and many states also require the approval of social service agencies.

There are two ways couples go about adopting a child: through an agency or privately. Licensed agencies oversee the entire adoption process, from the care of the birth mother to the screening of prospective parents to the placement of the child. Adoption agencies generally have long waiting lists.

Private adoptions bypass much of the agency bureaucracy, and much of the wait, as well. They are arranged by individuals, often an attorney who specializes in adoption, who bring together the woman who wants to place her baby with a couple who wants a child. The adoptive parents usually pay the birth mother's medical expenses and other related costs, but *they may not pay her to give up her child.* This is known as a "black market adoption," and it is illegal in every state.

Adoption is a complicated, lengthy process that can be fraught with disappointment and legal entanglements, as recently publicized court cases have shown. Seek expert legal counsel before you even begin, so you are fully aware of all the rights and risks involved. (See the Appendix for ways to acquire more information on adoption.)

Child Support and Alimony

"No area of family law is more rapidly changing or being more carefully scrutinized than the collective issues involved in alimony awards, child support, and child custody," says Sarah D. Eldrich, a marital attorney and chair of the Connecticut Bar Association Family Law Section. "New laws seek to impose uniform guidelines for child support and to nationalize enforcement policies, and there's an increasing awareness and concern about the effects of divorce on children, so much so that some states are now requiring parenting plans and parent education programs as part of the divorce proceedings when minor children are involved."

What all this means is that if either of you has been married before, any alimony and child support obligations you may have are not to be taken lightly. While alimony generally ceases when the recipient remarries, if one of you is paying alimony to an unmarried former spouse, that is not likely to change; alterations in child custody arrangements are even less likely to change. In fact, the only way these court determinations are usually modified is when some interested party petitions the court claiming "significantly altered circumstances."

The high rate of failure of noncustodial parents to meet their child-support obligations has become so scandalous that, starting in 1994, all child-support orders will require automatic wage deductions unless the parties have agreed otherwise or unless a court waives the order. Under the Child Support Recovery Act of 1992, it is now a federal offense to willfully neglect payment of support for over a year (or over the amount of $5,000) for a child residing in another state. That crime can be punished with fines and imprisonment.

One spouse's share of joint property cannot be attached to meet the alimony or child support obligations of the other, but liens can be placed on the jointly owned property. Thus, your lifestyle, and your property, can still be substantially affected by your spouse's obligations. If, for instance, a court rendered a judgment that necessitated the sale of your house in order to attach your spouse's share of that asset, or if a salary or an income tax refund were garnished, that would directly affect you. So, really, it is in your own best interest to help your spouse meet whatever obligations he or she may have.

If you didn't do so before this marriage, legal counsel is especially recommended now to preserve the inheritance rights and financial assets of any children from a former marriage and to safeguard any jointly owned property the two of you have accumulated. You might also want to review the terms of the divorce decree, especially if there are some enduring restrictions.

Marital Intervention

For far too long, law enforcement officials and government agencies maintained a hands-off policy on domestic interference. In the last decade or so, thanks to a growing number of crisis intervention services, protective shelters, help hot lines, community support groups, and, yes, a few well-publicized tragedies that could have been averted had law enforcement not failed to act, there is now more help and support available for victims of family violence and abuse.

In a situation of physical or emotional violence or drug or alcohol abuse between spouses, you have no more rights than any other individual in a similar situation, but at least you no longer have fewer rights. Here are the basic rights of self-protection you have under almost all state laws:

- To flee the abuser without it being considered desertion;
- To defend yourself with "reasonable force" when in eminent danger;
- To seek protection from a social service agency, the police, a shelter, or a church;
- To call the police;
- To file criminal charges;
- To testify voluntarily against a spouse in court;
- To file for a separation/divorce.

Here are additional rights you have in some states under what are being called "expanded domestic violence" laws:

- To have the abusive spouse removed from the house, at least temporarily;
- To file a civil suit for damages;
- To bring action for emotional pain;
- To charge a spouse with rape.

Unfortunately, you have no right, as a loving spouse, to involuntarily commit your husband or wife to a drug, alcohol, or mental health treatment center when the situation has gotten out of hand. The aid of an attending physician can be enlisted, however, because doctors do have legal authority, even a legal obligation, to intervene when a patient is a danger to himself or others. (See Appendix for hot-line information.)

Finding Legal Help

There are nearly 750,000 lawyers in the United States, so there must be one who's right for you out there somewhere. Most of the time, couples will initially contact a lawyer for a routine need, such as drafting a will, closing on a house, reviewing a contract, or some other ordinary, uncomplicated chore. The lawyer you contact for one need may or may not become "your lawyer" for other matters. That will depend on you and on the attorney's area of expertise.

If you have serious complications, for example, if you've been charged with a crime, then obviously, the attorney's expertise in the practice of criminal law would be of paramount importance. Seventeen states have instituted what are called "specialization programs." These programs provide some form of certification for attorneys to practice in a specific area, such as domestic relations or tax law, thereby assuring specialized knowledge and experience in a field.

You can check with your state bar association to find out if your state is one offering specialization programs and, if so, what they are. In states without specializations, you might want to ask your attorney what he or she considers to be a particular area of legal expertise or concentration. Most lawyers will make referrals to a colleague when they feel a client's needs indicate more specialized knowledge (and they do not charge referral fees).

The best referral is always a personal one, a recommendation from a friend or family members. If you're new to a community and don't know anyone whose recommendation you'd trust, you can contact the professional associations. Some state bar associations have referral services, but many do not. Local and regional bar associations are much more likely to make referrals, from among their own membership.

Bar association membership is required in some states and voluntary in others, but participation in professional organizations can always be taken as a good indication of one's credibility and acceptance in the legal community. (See the list of state bar associations at the end of this chapter.) In addition to referrals, most state and local associations make available client information on a variety of subjects, including legal services, housing, small claims court, and myriad other topics. The American Bar Association, too, offers information and publications to the general public on general legal matters (see Appendix).

If you can't afford a private attorney, there are legal assistance programs in most communities. Legal aid offices may have their own staff of lawyers or they may use volunteer attorneys. Usually, you'll have to meet certain guidelines (income level, residency requirements) to become eligible for free or reduced-fee services. Look under legal aid in the phone book, or contact the county courthouse, the district attorney's office, or the local or state bar association to find out more about legal assistance programs.

However you go about finding an attorney, the American Bar Association suggests you have a preliminary meeting before you actually retain a lawyer's services, especially for a serious matter. Some questions to consider when evaluating whether or not a particular attorney is right for you appear in the following box. (For a more complete American Bar Association guide to choosing an attorney, see the Appendix).

Questions to Ask about Legal Representation

1. What is this lawyer's particular area of expertise in legal practice?
2. Who (this attorney, an associate, a paralegal, or a clerk) will be handling my case/affairs?
3. How are fees charged and what is the billing procedure?
4. Does this attorney seem willing, and able, to answer my questions and to offer me the kind of advice and representation I need?
5. Is this attorney sufficiently accessible (location, office hours, staff, messages) to meet my needs?

State Bar Associations

Courtesy American Bar Association

Alabama State Bar
P.O. Box 671
Montgomery, AL 36101
205/269-1515

Alaska Bar Association
P.O. Box 100279
Anchorage, AK 99510
907/272-7469

State Bar of Arizona
363 N. 1st Ave.
Phoenix, AZ 85003
602/252-4804

Arkansas Bar Association
400 W. Markham
Little Rock, AR 72201
501/375-4605

State Bar of California
555 Franklin St.
San Francisco, CA 94102
415/561-8200

The Colorado Bar Association
1900 Grant St. #950
Denver, CO 80203
303/860-1115

Connecticut Bar Association
101 Corporate Pl.
Rocky Hill, CT 06067
203/721-0025

Delaware State Bar Association
1225 King St.
Wilmington, DE 19801
302/658-5279

Bar Association of the
    District of Columbia
1819 H St., NW
12th Floor
Washington, DC 20006-3690
202/223-6600

The District of Columbia Bar
1707 L St., NW
6th Floor
Washington, DC 20036
202/331-3883

The Florida Bar
650 Apalachee Pkwy.
Tallahassee, FL 32399-2300
904/561-5600

State Bar of Georgia
800 The Hurt Bldg.
50 Hurt Plaza
Atlanta, GA 30303
404/527-8700

Hawaii State Bar Association
1136 Union Mall
Honolulu, HI 96813
808/537-1868

Idaho State Bar
P.O. Box 895
Boise, ID 83701
208/342-8958

Illinois State Bar Association
424 S. Second St.
Springfield, IL 62701
217/525-1760

Indiana State Bar Association
230 E. Ohio, 4th Fl.
Indianapolis, IN 46204
317/639-5465

The Iowa State Bar Association
521 E. Locust
Des Moines, IA 50309
515/243-3179

Kansas Bar Association
P.O. Box 1037
Topeka, KS 66601-1037
913/234-5696

Kentucky Bar Association
514 W. Main St.
Frankfort, KY 40601-1883
502/564-3795

Louisiana State Bar Association
601 St. Charles Ave.
New Orleans, LA 70130
504/566-1600

Maine State Bar Association
P.O. Box 788
Augusta, ME 04332-0788
207/622-7523

Maryland State Bar Association, Inc.
520 W. Fayette St.
Baltimore, MD 21201
410/685-7878

Massachusetts Bar Association
20 West St.
Boston, MA 02111
617/542-3602

State Bar of Michigan
306 Townsend St.
Lansing, MI 48933-2083
517/372-9030

Minnesota State Bar Association
514 Nicollet Mall
Suite 300
Minneapolis, MN 55402
612/333-1183

The Mississippi State Bar
P.O. Box 2168
Jackson, MS 39225-2168
601/948-4471

The Missouri Bar
P.O. Box 119
Jefferson City, MO 65102
314/635-4128

State Bar of Montana
P.O. Box 577
Helena, MT 59624
406/442-7660

Nebraska State Bar Association
P.O. Box 81809
Lincoln, NE 68501
402/475-7091

State Bar of Nevada
201 Las Vegas Blvd.
Suite 200
Las Vegas, NV 89101
702/382-2200

New Hampshire Bar Association
112 Pleasant St.
Concord, NH 03301
603/224-6942

New Jersey State Bar Association
New Jersey Law Center
One Constitution Sqr.
New Brunswick, NJ 08901-1500
908/249-5000

State Bar of New Mexico
P.O. Box 25883
Albuquerque, NM 87125
505/842-6132

New York State Bar Association
One Elk St.
Albany, NY 12207
518/463-3200

North Carolina State Bar
P.O. Box 25908
Raleigh, NC 27611
919/828-4620

North Carolina Bar Association
P.O. Box 12806
Raleigh, NC 27605
919/828-0561

State Bar Association of
    North Dakota
515½ E. Broadway
Suite 101
Bismarck, ND 58502
701/255-1404

Ohio State Bar Association
P.O. Box 16562
Columbus, OH 43216-6562
614/487-2050

Oklahoma Bar Association
P.O. Box 53036
Oklahoma City, OK 73152
405/524-2365

Oregon State Bar
P.O. Box 1689
Lake Oswego, OR 97035
503/620-0222

Pennsylvania Bar Association
P.O. Box 186
Harrisburg, PA 17108
717/238-6715

Puerto Rico Bar Association
P.O. Box 1900
San Juan, PR 00903
809/721-3358

Rhode Island Bar Association
115 Cedar St.
Providence, RI 02903
401/421-5740

South Carolina Bar
P.O. Box 608
Columbia, SC 29202
803/799-6653

State Bar of South Dakota
222 E. Capitol
Pierre, SD 57501
605/224-7554

Tennessee Bar Association
3622 West End Ave.
Nashville, TN 37205
615/383-7421

State Bar of Texas
P.O. Box 12487
Austin, TX 78711
512/463-1400

Utah State Bar
645 S. 200 East, #310
Salt Lake City, UT 84111
801/531-9077

Vermont Bar Association
P.O. Box 100
Montpelier, VT 05601
802/223-2020

Virginia State Bar
707 E. Main St.
Suite 1500
Richmond, VA 23219-2803
804/775-0500

Virginia Bar Association
7th & Franklin Bldg.
701 E. Franklin St. #1515
Richmond, VA 23219
804/644-0041

Virgin Islands Bar Association
P.O. Box 4108
Christiansted, VI 00822
809/778-7497

Washington State Bar Association
500 Westin Bldg.
2001 6th Ave.
Seattle, WA 98121-2599
206/727-8200

West Virginia Bar Association
P.O. Box 346
Charleston, WV 25322
304/342-1474

West Virginia State Bar
2006 Kanawha Blvd. E.
Charleston, WV 25311
304/558-2456

State Bar of Wisconsin
402 W. Wilson
Madison, WI 53703
608/257-3838

Wyoming State Bar
P.O. Box 109
Cheyenne, WY 82003-0109
307/632-9061

CHAPTER 11
Staying Healthy

M arriage is a new beginning, and new beginnings are good for the soul. You may have noticed it already, the invigorating energy love has brought to your life. You are filled with positive impulses, and eager to meet the challenges of each new day. There is simply nothing the two of you are afraid to tackle—together.

New beginnings can also be good for the body, especially when you strive to look and act as well as you feel. After all, good health is more than an absence of sickness. It's a state of integrated well-being, a fitness of body, mind, and spirit. The more sophisticated and technological we get in the treatment and diagnosis of illness, the more we can use simple reminders on how to treat ourselves well.

Sound nutrition, regular exercise, reduced stress, occasional relaxation, satisfying work, meaningful relationships, and regular preventative healthcare— these measures not only help to ward off disease, but they help preserve and protect the "total wellness" that should be your goal. As newlyweds, you will probably spend a lot of time sharing your dreams and shaping your plans for the future. You'll want to do all you can to ensure a long and healthy life ahead in which to pursue them.

Today, because of extensive health care research and fitness awareness, we know just how much of our quality of life depends on our own ability to develop healthful habits within a reasonably balanced lifestyle. That knowledge can be empowering. With it, we can assume more responsibility for our own health and happiness.

Can Happiness Be Hazardous to Your Health?

Fact: most newlyweds gain weight the first year of marriage. Why? Because they rely on convenience products and take-out meals to compensate for hectic schedules, or because they build their social lives around food, or because their bodies simply respond to a change in diet and eating habits.

✨ Do You See Yourself Here? ✨

- Have you noticed any dramatic change in your eating, drinking, or sleeping habits since you've been married?
- Has one of you gained, or lost, a significant amount of weight?
- Do you realize that you know very little about nutrition and health?
- Have you let your regular exercise regimen slip?
- Are you under considerably more stress now that you're married than you were when you were single?
- Have you failed to be as attentive to your physical appearance as you were before you were married?
- Has a combination of poor health habits and careless personal attention caused your self-esteem to falter?
- Have you let regular health checkups slide, thereby jeopardizing preventative health care?
- Does either of you exhibit any danger signs of dependencies or psychological disorders?

Read on for remedies to those "yes" answers.

Sometimes newlyweds get carried away by the sheer fun of shopping and cooking together. "When I was single," says Samantha, now married only a little over a year, "I didn't prepare elaborate meals for myself. I ate simply, but well: lots of fresh fruit and vegetables, salads, yogurt, cereal, broiled chicken or fish. Now, I still have those things in the house, but somehow, my eating and cooking habits have changed considerably."

Marriage has changed them. Like many lucky couples, Samantha and Serge had a large wedding and received some lovely gifts, among them a microwave oven, a food processor, a barbecue grill, complete sets of cookware and cutlery, and numerous small appliances, cookbooks, and kitchen gadgets. Overwhelmed by the culinary possibilities and eager to share a new interest and activity, they became, in Serge's words, "instant gourmets."

"Food became more than a hobby for us," explains Samantha, "it became a passion. Exotic dishes, fine wines, entertaining in style—every experiment was a new adventure. Sure we were gaining weight, but we shrugged it off as being happily married people."

But when Samantha could no longer wear her most expensive dinner dress and Serge could no longer button his favorite blazer, they weren't so happy. They knew that 15 pounds overweight the first year would turn into 30 the next unless they curbed this great culinary adventure. They would have to redirect their knowledge about food selection and preparation toward more balanced, sensible eating habits. But first, they had to reevaluate the role food played in their lives and then learn to plan accordingly.

Settling Down and Settling In

Marriage makes a dramatic difference in your life. Suddenly there's another person to consider. You have to adjust to each other's eating habits, sleeping patterns, and work and play routines. As a couple, you may have hectic schedules and busy social lives. You probably entertain more, find yourselves with more business and family obligations, and yearn for more time to spend at home together. You discover that being a couple is a lot more demanding than being single.

In the process of adapting to a new situation, it's easy to fall into bad habits without even thinking about them. Sometimes, we don't even see the behaviors as bad, but just new and different. Unless something forces us into awareness of just how harmful they are, these bad habits can easily stay with us for the rest of our lives.

Don't let that happen to you. Now is a good time to examine your overall lifestyle from a health perspective. A change in circumstances, more than simply being married, can precipitate the different routines and behaviors that, in turn, affect your physical and mental health. Moving from a rural area to a city, for instance, can mean more dinners out or a change in exercise levels. A new job with longer hours can mean interrupted mealtimes, more stress, or changes in sleep patterns. If you don't modify your habits to compensate for these new routines, you can easily gain weight, get out of shape, become irritable and depressed, or otherwise erode the good health, and the healthy outlook, you brought to marriage.

You need to take a realistic look at the changes in routines that marriage has brought, and to resolve to make whatever adjustments are needed in your behaviors. Samantha and Serge began by analyzing their lifestyle and admitting that they were somewhat sedentary to begin with. They sat at their jobs, they sat on the train to commute, they sat at movies and theater, they sat to read a book. Maybe instead of cooking such elaborate meals in the evening, they should use some of the extra time to take a walk or ride their bikes and get some much needed exercise. Then, too, since both were executives and had frequent business lunches and dinner engagements, they really didn't need to be having such big meals at home every night anyway.

The couple agreed to make an effort to find other activities, particularly more physically active ones, that they could enjoy besides cooking and eating: cultural events, sure, but also sports, outdoor recreation, yard work and home-improvement projects.

When the couple did cook and entertain, mostly on weekends, they challenged themselves to find ways to adapt their favorite, fancy recipes to sensible, low-fat, low-cholesterol dishes that would present just as beautifully and deliciously. During the week, they rediscovered Samantha's premarriage preferences for fresh fruits, salads, yogurt, and simply grilled meats for quick, healthy dinners at home.

What Other Couples Say . . .

Changes in lifestyle after marriage often have positive effects, especially when you marry a more health-conscious partner. Couples regularly say, with pride, that one of them has helped the other eat more balanced meals, or get more involved in sports and fitness, or adjust their attitudes in stressful situations. In repeated studies, married people consistently report better physical and psychological health than their unmarried cohorts.

Randy, a newlywed who lowered his cholesterol level, lost a few pounds, and actually learned to like exercise during his first year of marriage to a slim, trim, "nutrition freak," admits he's never looked or felt better in his life. "Everyone should get married," he says. "It's good for you!"

Nutritional Know-How

Shopping and planning for balanced meals may take a little extra time and effort in the beginning, particularly if you don't know as much as you'd like about basic nutrition. The food industry is a big business and, while the government requires that suppliers list nutritional information on their packages, some of that information can be pretty obscure and misleading as well.

Oddly, even well-intentioned nutritional research often adds to the confusion. While much of this research is valuable and important, the general public is perhaps too quick to interpret preliminary findings as absolute fact. We leap to unfounded conclusions, such as all fats are bad, or that vitamin E improves one's sex life, or that a particular nutrient can prevent or cure a certain disease. Then, when conflicting data emerges later, we don't know what to believe.

The best principle, and the only one on which virtually all nutritionists agree, is just common sense: a balance and a variety of food intake will enhance the pleasure and minimize the potential harm any one food could do. Unless you have some particular food allergies that you're aware of, the best bet might be to look again at the old "basic food groups" chart from your high-school health text.

Actually, there are many more excellent books and reference materials available to help you learn what you need to know about food selection and preparation. There are even computer software programs to help you plan meals and track calories, fats, carbohydrates, etc. The American Heart Association offers numerous booklets and pamphlets on cooking and eating right (see Appendix), and their specialty cookbooks are readily available in bookstores.

While you're learning more about healthful eating, start to build better nutritional habits right now with these quick and easy tips:

- Be adventuresome. Why limit salads to ho-hum iceberg lettuce, for instance, when there are also chard, chicory, endive, kale, collards, and a variety of cabbages to choose from? Be willing to try new things.

- Be creative in the use of spices and natural sugars to perk up the flavor of food. Chicken with tarragon doesn't need table salt; herbal tea with lemon doesn't need processed sugar. Experiment. When foods are seasoned properly, you won't be tempted to reach for the sugar bowl or salt shaker.
- Eat slowly. Slower eating aids in digestion, allows you to enjoy your food more, and results in eating less.
- Make choices. Vowing to never have an ice cream sundae again is unreasonable, and probably impossible, but you can learn to make trade-offs. Have the sundae as a weekend treat, but only once a month. Have dessert at lunch, but not at dinner, or make a choice between a buttered roll or sour cream on your baked potato at the same meal. Choices like these will give you greater dietary variety while allowing you to maintain weight control on a continuing basis without feeling deprived.
- Be a smart partygiver and partygoer. As hosts, make sure there's something being offered for everyone, even those watching their weight. Fruits and vegetables make attractive nibbles and side dishes; dips and sauces made with yogurt, margarine, and other less fatty ingredients are a welcome accompaniment. Avoid salty foods, as they encourage guests to drink more, and never insist that someone eat or drink more than he wants.
- As a guest, have a nutritious snack before you leave home, especially if you know there will be a long cocktail hour with lots of fatty foods ahead. Choose tall drinks made with soda, seltzer, or water so they last longer, and position yourself for conversation away from the buffet table or bar.
- Shop and cook together. Food, its preparation, presentation, and consumption, is one of life's true pleasures, and it's a pleasure couples can share. Make your meals together really special by planning menus that are attractive, palate pleasing, and good for each of you. Just think of it as another way to show you care.

Dieting the Healthy Way

Statistics show that 95 percent of those who lose weight on a "quick loss" diet scheme gain it back within two years. Renata is typical. Eager to be a superslim bride, she lost 15 pounds on a crash diet in one month before her wedding. Before her first anniversary, she had gained all the weight, and then some, back. "I was so disgusted with myself," she recalls. "I didn't know what to do next. It was depressing."

Like so many women, Renata has been off and on every conceivable diet there is since adolescence. Over the years this dieting-binging syndrome produced a yo-yo effect on her weight that was not only personally frustrating, but physically dangerous. To make matters worse, her new husband, Cal, has no weight problem whatsoever.

"The prospect of dieting once again was dismal enough," Renata recalls, "but to face dieting while Cal was eating as much as he wanted made it that much more discouraging."

Fifteen Food Facts or Fallacies

How Much Do You Know?

Try taking this test together to see how much you really know.

1. A four-ounce serving of halibut has more protein and less fat than the same size serving of prime rib.	True False
2. We can substitute tea, coffee, or other beverages for our eight glasses of water a day.	True False
3. There is no harm in adult consumption of one or two alcoholic beverages a day.	True False
4 The body's protein requirements decrease with age.	True False
5. Smaller, more frequent meals are better than three meals a day.	True False
6. If something is good for you, more of it must be better.	True False
7. No single food contains all the nutrients the body needs.	True False
8. Heavy doses of vitamin C will prevent colds.	True False
9. A potato and a carrot contain approximately the same calories.	True False
10. Most of us do need some sort of vitamin/mineral supplements.	True False
11. Meat, fish, and poultry contain fiber.	True False
12. Milk (or skim milk) is as important for adults as children.	True False
13. Raw vegetables are always better for you than cooked.	True False
14. "Natural" or "organic" foods are superior to foods you buy in supermarkets.	True False
15. A simple switch from saturated (lard, meat fat, butter, whole milk) to polyunsaturated fats (vegetable oils, fish, poultry, skim milk) can reduce harmful blood cholesterol levels.	True False

Answers: True: 1, 3, 4, 5, 7, 9, 12, and 15
False: 2, 6, 8, 10, 11, 13, and 14

Good for you if you got more than ten right. If "you are what you eat," you must be a 10! Remember your food facts, and you'll stay that way.

Luckily for her, Renata's dilemma brought her to the right conclusion: fad diets don't work. The only way anyone can lose weight safely and hope to keep it off is to reduce the caloric intake and increase exercise. A weight loss goal of two pounds a week is reasonable. The only way to keep the weight off, though, is to permanently modify behavior. You can't go back to being a couch potato, and eating potatoes—French fried or with sour cream or butter or gravy—at every meal, and expect to maintain your new weight.

Renata began to jog with Cal in the morning, shorter distances at first, and started taking the stairs or the long way whenever she could. By doing a little nutritional homework, she soon discovered that she could have most of the same foods Cal enjoyed, but in smaller portions. She has also learned to make wise choices, such as substituting the natural sugar of fruits for the artificial sugar of candy bars to get her through her late-afternoon energy slump.

Renata is looking and feeling great these days, and for the first time in her adult life, has achieved a balanced diet and exercise program she can live with. "I think Cal is a lot happier, too," she confesses, "because I don't have all this craziness about food anymore. We're out enjoying things together and life is normal—and fun."

If either of you has a weight problem, take a lesson from Renata. Forget the fads and adhere to the basic principle of thermodynamics: reduce intake and increase activity. Start off by determining your ideal weight, and then set a reasonable time frame in which to achieve it. Enlist your spouse's help to strengthen your resolve so that by dieting the right way, once and for all, you won't have to keep on dieting forever, moving from one fad fix to the next.

Two points before we leave the subject of dieting: first of all, overweight is defined as being 10 percent over your ideal weight, and obesity is defined as 20 percent. But only you know what your ideal weight, the weight at which you look, feel, and perform at your best, really is. The charts you see in doctors' offices and fitness centers are fine as guidelines, but they may not apply to your individual health circumstances and body characteristics. Be realistic and be reasonable. Studies have shown that constant fluctuations in weight, due to unreasonable expectations, can actually be more detrimental to health than being somewhat overweight.

Secondly, while a healthy self-image is certainly related to looking well and being satisfied with what you see in the mirror, obsessing over every pound is not normal, and an undue preoccupation with food, eating either too much or too little of it, presages a full-blown eating disorder. If your relationship with food seems to indicate the need for some professional counseling, get it. Eating should be a pleasure, not a source of guilt and pain.

Move Those Bodies

If you don't take care of your body, where are you going to live? This is a favorite quip of fitness fanatics as they pull, push, and prod their bodies into perfect proportions while some of us sit on the sidelines, in sedentary fashion, and watch. In defense of our inactivity, perhaps, we are quick to point out the dangers of bodily stress and the illnesses and injuries that can be caused by too much exercise.

As in most other things, balance and common sense are key to any successful fitness program. Exercise is not a panacea. It will not, in and of itself, cure disease, prolong life, or make you beautiful. But it will, in combination with other healthful habits, keep the body you have looking, feeling, and performing at its best.

Again, forget crackpot claims and compulsive competition. The overwhelming consensus of scientific and medical opinion supports two basic conclusions: the real benefits of regular, reasonable exercise are long-term and preventative in nature, and Americans, in general, do not integrate enough physical activity into their daily routines. As newlyweds, your commitment to fitness is an insurance policy for the future because what you do for yourselves today will pay dividends in the years to come.

The two of you don't have to be the most athletic couple on the block. In fact, athletic prowess is largely an inherited characteristic anyway. Even if watching the Olympics is the closest you can come to mustering an enthusiasm for sports, there are ways to be among the fittest viewers.

Choosing a Fitness Regimen

When examining your attitudes about fitness and health, it is important to recognize your limitations and to identify personal goals. As with diet plans, no one fitness program is right for everybody. As a couple, each of you has different needs, and maybe different preferences. The trick is to find a way to dovetail those needs and preferences.

Kate and Marvin are a classic example of the old adage, "opposites attract." Marvin is the outdoor, athletic type. Long before he was married, he jogged, played softball, and worked out at the gym at lunchtime. He still does. Kate, on the other hand, is an avid reader, a devotee of the opera and the ballet, and a consummate homemaker who enjoys mostly indoor pursuits, such as sewing and crafts projects. While each always took pride in the other's skills and accomplishments, each also realized after marriage that they needed to spend more time together in activities they could both enjoy.

Fully aware of her tendency toward a sedentary lifestyle, Kate suggested after-dinner walks as a simple way to spend some time together while increasing her own level of physical activity. These walks turned into walk-talks, and during one of them, Marvin invited her down to see the gym where he worked out. "What a discovery that was!" Kate says now. "It wasn't a smelly old gym at all, but a sleek, modern fitness center with all sorts of interesting activities worth investigating."

Now, three times a week, Kate and Marvin meet at "the gym." He does his body building and she does aerobic dancing—to classical music, no less. On Saturdays, after their sessions, they often seek out unusual spots for a leisurely lunch or picnic. Their walk-talks in the evenings have continued, but they have gotten brisker, eliminating Marvin's desire to jog. "I feel like we're not only keeping ourselves in shape," Kate says, "but we're keeping our marriage in shape, too."

Fitness facts are not complicated and exercise opportunities are not limited to the sports arena. When we integrate a fitness awareness into the total context of our daily routines and interests, we might discover, as Kate and Marvin have, that satisfying the body's need for exercise can produce benefits that go beyond the strictly physical.

Assessing Your Fitness Potential

Those who are fit and active enjoy:

- Reduced risks of cardiovascular disease
- Stronger musculoskeletal systems
- Better weight control
- Increased energy and stamina
- Heightened feelings of well-being
- Reduced anxiety and increased self-esteem

Now that's a lot of benefit for as little physical exercise as 20 minutes a day or 45 minutes three times a week. The trick is to be steady and regular in your pattern of weekly exercise, and to choose enough variety in physical activity to satisfy the body's many movement needs.

There are three aspects of physical fitness: flexibility, strength, and endurance. Some exercises concentrate more on one aspect, like weight lifting to build strength and tone muscles, while other activities, such as aerobic dancing, are designed to develop all three. It doesn't matter so much which specific exercise(s) you do so long as you choose one, or a combination of several, that meet multiple body needs.

Most of all, whether you want to get in shape or want to get in better shape, remember that flexibility, strength, and endurance are built slowly, a step at a time. Don't ever forget the all-important warm-up and cool-down periods recommended before and after every session, and always remember that too much too soon may be dangerous. (See Appendix for exercise guidelines from the American Heart Association.)

Seven Ways to Shape Up

1. Analyze your interest and lifestyle. Most exercise dropouts occur because enthusiasm wanes or time constraints prevail. If you choose an activity that you enjoy and that can be easily integrated into your schedule, you are twice as likely to stick to it.
2. Investigate before you begin. Not all fitness programs are equal. Verify the quality of supervision, equipment, facilities, etc., before committing yourself to any club or fitness center, and be sure you like the activity before investing in expensive paraphernalia.

3. Know your physical condition and limitations. An examination by a physician is a good idea before beginning any new fitness program. This is vital if you have a history of cardiovascular problems or muscular or skeletal injuries or ailments. A checkup is also advised for those in high health-risk categories such as heavy smokers, the obese, diabetics, or those with other chronic health conditions that must be monitored.

4. Utilize expert resources. Besides your doctor, you may also have access to referral sources at your local hospital, health clubs, or the YMCA/YWCA. Through them, you can get stress tests, fitness assessments, and professional advice on what programs and activities suit you. Often, exercise physiologists are available on site to give expert advice.

5. Start slowly and don't overdo. Other than the most minor aches from renewed use of long-neglected muscles, there should be no real, lasting pain associated with proper exercise. Strain and injury occur when the body is pushed beyond reasonable limits, or when too much is attempted too soon. Anyone who tells you that good exercise is supposed to hurt is wrong.

6. Listen to your body. Learn to become attuned to your body rhythms and exercise at your own pace. Pay attention to physical symptoms of stress and fatigue (dizziness, shortness of breath, sudden pain, etc.) and be sensible in your expectations of yourself, particularly if you haven't been physically active for a long time.

7. Use fitness activities to get in shape for a sport, not the other way around. Games like tennis, squash, racketball, and the like are not for unconditioned beginners. When and if you decide to pursue a sport, be sure that you're in adequate physical condition to undertake it, and that you have sufficient instruction and appropriate equipment so as to avoid a mishap or injury.

Preventative Health Care

The name of the game in health care is prevention and early detection. You each should have had a complete physical before your wedding. If not, take care of that now. Routine medical checkups need to be part of your regular health and fitness routine, for both of you. It is helpful to schedule your checkups around important dates, birthdays or anniversaries, so it's easy to remember when they're due. (Your regular doctors and dentists can also send you reminders in the mail if you ask them to do so.)

The frequency and extent to which a healthy person should be examined by a health-care professional is always a matter of some discussion and debate. Your own health history and health risks, plus the advice of your particular doctor, are the best guides. Nevertheless, here are some general guidelines from the major health associations:

• The Report of the U.S. Preventive Services Task Force (1989), which is endorsed by the American Medical Association, recommends that adults between the ages of 19 and 39 have general physical examinations every one to three years, depending on their inclusion in certain high-risk categories. The physical should include checks on weight and blood pressure, as well as routine laboratory/diagnostic procedures.

- The American College of Obstetricians and Gynecologists advocates yearly gynecologic exams and Pap tests, and monthly self breast examinations. Mammograms should be scheduled regularly, at a frequency determined by you and your doctor.
- The American Dental Association recommends professional cleaning, polishing, and dental checkups on a regular basis to prevent periodontal disease. Your dentist will tell you how often you should visit, but in between visits, you can practice preventative dentistry by thoroughly brushing and flossing twice a day, and by eating a balanced diet. (See Appendix for more information on dental care.)
- The American Optometric Association recommends eye exams for adults every one to two years. People in high-risk categories for developing eye strain or glaucoma should follow their optometrist's/ophthalmologist's advice on how often to schedule checkups. (See Appendix for more information.)

Finding Health Services

If you've moved to a new city, you'll have to locate a doctor, dentist, gynecologist, optometrist or ophthalmologist, and maybe a veterinarian for your pet, as well as any other specialist you might need. Sometimes, a former physician can recommend a doctor in your new location; otherwise, you can check directories in the library or get listings from local hospitals, clinics, or professional medical associations. These sources will not provide you with recommendations. They will only give you the names of license holders, membership listings, or practitioners in specific areas.

Most of us rely on word-of-mouth recommendations from neighbors and friends, and that is probably the best bet. But don't wait until you have a medical emergency to find a doctor, dentist, or other health professional. Secure one in advance, make an appointment just to meet the person, and have your health records forwarded. (It's also not a bad idea to locate the nearest hospital emergency room, either, just in case.)

On your initial visit, don't be shy about asking questions. Choosing a physician is an important step in your own health-care choices, and you want to feel that a trusting, understanding relationship is likely to grow between you. During your first office visit, you need to find out about:

- What's included in fees and services and what might be billed separately
- How fees are to be paid and what the procedures are for insurance reimbursement

- What services will be referred elsewhere (such as routine blood tests, x rays, etc.)
- What hospital or clinic this professional uses
- Who will cover when this doctor is unavailable
- The convenience of office hours and how emergency situations are handled

The American Medical Association offers a consumer guide, complete with questions to ask, called "Choosing Your Physician." (See Appendix.)

Positive Persuasions

"I am so-o-o-o stressed out!" How many times a day do we hear that, say that, witness that in action? Stress. It's what everybody talks about and worries about. Sometimes, it's even used as an excuse for unreasonable behavior.

"I really was stressed," Bobbie explains. "I mean, I had school, and the job, and a sick mother, and I felt like the whole world was on my shoulders. The more I got into feeling sorry for myself, the more I expected Mike to cater to me."

Mike didn't take much to catering, though, and so the couple found themselves in repeated conflict over stupid, little things. "One night, when we started arguing over which spoon to stir the spaghetti sauce with, I thought, now this is really ridiculous," Bobbie recalls. "In fact, it was more than ridiculous. It was humiliating."

Over the spaghetti sauce, Mike finally let it all out. He told Bobbie that she had become totally self-absorbed in her own problems and her own self, that nothing, not even her mother's illness was that serious, and that he was tired of hearing about her stressed-out life. "Everybody deals with stress," he told her. "Grow up!"

Luckily for both of them, Bobbie was in the mood to hear what he said and took note. She realized how much of her daily aggravations she was taking out on Mike, and how good-natured he had been to put up with her self-indulgent "stressing" for so long. She had been unfair, and she knew it. Admitting this to Mike was perhaps the most important thing she could do, for both of them.

Most of the time, it isn't a major problem that gets us down; rather, it is the cumulative effect of everyday coping with minor nuisances—boredom, inefficiency, insecurity, inconvenience—that gets to us. We lose our patience, and our temper, and ultimately our equilibrium, over something insignificant, like spoons for stirring the spaghetti sauce.

We've already talked about all sorts of stresses elsewhere in this book, about its many sources and what we might do to mitigate its effects in various situations. Let's not forget, either, that stress is not always bad. It is, after all, the motivation that gets the old adrenaline going and pushes the winner across the finish line.

As a rule, it's the way we perceive the challenges in our lives, rather than the challenges themselves, that causes a positive or a negative reaction to the stressor. When we start to feel victimized by everything, "stressing out" becomes a way of life, as it did for Bobbie. That's a dangerous way to live, because constant, uninterrupted tension can lead to serious physical and emotional problems. And it doesn't do much to enhance your relationships either.

De-Stressing

We all have our hang-ups and nobody's perfect, but we can mitigate the effects of daily stress in our lives with some basic, commonsense approaches. Mostly, it's a matter of cultivating some "presence of mind," some collectedness, before reacting prematurely to people and situations around us. Here are some suggestions to help you get in control.

- Get adequate rest, especially when you know you're about to enter a period of stress in your life. It's hard to handle even simple situations when you're overtired.
- Talk to yourself and bolster your own self-esteem. Instead of concentrating on what you haven't accomplished or don't have, why not make a list of what you have done or do have? You might be surprised at its length.
- When you feel overwhelmed, take some time out to set priorities. Then, begin slowly, start with the least appealing task first, and remind yourself that everything will get done, one step at a time.
- Talk about your dreams and goals. This verbal visualization technique is not only healthy, but it is a proven confidence builder, especially if you have someone you love who shares your dreams.
- Allow yourself to vent emotions. You have a right to experience honest feelings of sadness, anger, happiness, and silliness, and to express them. But then, when you have, that's it.
- Practice simple relaxation techniques. Just a deep breath or five minutes of pleasant daydreams with eyes closed can do wonders.
- Lift sagging spirits with a few minutes of vigorous exercise. This will also give you some time to think and to get back in touch with yourself. Exercise may even release certain "feel good" chemicals in the brain.
- When all else fails, or even if it doesn't, laugh. There's nothing more therapeutic than humor.

Mind over Matter

We've often heard the response, when someone is complaining of anxiety or the blues or a minor physical ailment, "Oh, it's all in your head." Ironically, current scientific research on the relationship of brain chemistry to bodily functioning and emotional makeup would clearly support that conclusion.

The human being is a biological composite of body, mind, and spirit. This is the guiding philosophy of the holistic health approach, and of alternative medicine, and why more and more emphasis, even within the traditional medical establishment, is being placed on looking at the total person (mental, emotional, and physical) when treating disease or planning preventative health care. A positive mental attitude is integral to one's well-being; the ability to influence the way we feel and behave by the way we think may be the single greatest tool each of us has for achieving, and preserving, our own physical and mental health.

Now that the two of you are just beginning your new lives together, you have every reason to be optimistic and excited about your future. Yet, life is not easy, and stress and anxiety are commonplace in American society. There may be changes and disappointments, frustrations and failures, struggles and surprises, and you will have to cope, in a constructive, productive way. Even good news, unexpected windfalls, or exceptional good fortune can bring stressful adjustments.

People don't go in for routine mental health checkups the way they go for physical checkups, so bolstering each other and helping each other maintain a healthy attitude becomes a loving task the two of you will have to do for yourselves. Love, support, encouragement, humor, these are the ways you lighten life's burdens for each other, and most of the time they work.

But, sometimes the burdens get too great and the anxieties, fears, and depressions mount. A loved one can change through anger or violence, alcohol or drug abuse. One partner can become depressed, withdrawn, a virtual stranger. If one of you gets into emotional trouble, the other will have to have the courage to identify it as a mental health problem, and to insist that help be obtained.

Mental illness does not discriminate; it strikes at every age, race, and socioeconomic level. Estimates are that between 30 and 45 million Americans suffer from manifestations of a mental disorder or dependency that impairs their daily functioning to some extent. These disorders could be diagnosed and treated if only the people, or their loved ones on their behalf, would seek professional help.

If you or your spouse exhibit any of the danger signs of mental illness, don't jeopardize your future health and happiness because of outdated stereotypes and stigmas regarding mental health treatment. Get the help you need. Here, from the American Psychiatric Association, are the Ten Warning Signs of Mental Illness (see the Appendix for more information):

1. Marked personality change
2. Inability to cope with problems and daily activities
3. Strange or grandiose ideas
4. Excessive anxieties
5. Prolonged depression and apathy

6. Marked changes in eating or sleeping patterns
7. Thinking or talking about suicide
8. Extreme highs and lows
9. Abuse of alcohol or drugs
10. Excessive anger, hostility, or violent behavior

Health, and Beauty, Too

"Zest is the secret of all beauty," said Christian Dior. Being newly married and in love, you have zest in abundance right now. You'll want to hold onto it, and learn to use it to your best, most beautiful advantage.

Mother Nature will do a lot of beautifying for us if we will just work with her. A few minutes a day spent in routine personal care can maintain and maximize whatever we've got going for us in the first place, and regular attention to reasonable diet and exercise can keep us in optimum health and peak physical condition. These small efforts promote a habit of wellness and an overall sense of well-being.

When you're happy with yourself and proud of each other, you achieve a beauty and a vitality that won't fade with age.

It's called "a zest for life," and it shows.

CHAPTER 12

Celebrating the Future

Forty years ago, Jackie Gleason made television history with his famous sitcom, "The Honeymooners." Perhaps you've seen reruns. In case you haven't, let's be clear that we're not talking about a couple like Ozzie and Harriet, or even Lucy and Desi. No, Ralph and Alice Cramden were working-class people (he was a bus driver) who lived in a city apartment and had no children. Each week, American audiences watched the Cramdens struggling to make ends meet while also struggling to make sense of their lives.

"The Honeymooners" succeeded, and endured, precisely because that life didn't always make sense and was hardly idyllic; Gleason got his laughs at the expense of the small tragedies and harsh realities married couples faced every day. And so viewers shook their heads, chuckled with recognition, and were led to see the humor in their own predicaments.

If you watch "The Honeymooners" today, you may think the situations quaint or naive, the attitudes sexist or stereotypical, but you will find the show funny, in a tragi-comic way. The world view of the ancient Greeks still speaks to us. So, regardless of how crazy, or how stupid, or how hardheaded any of the characters might have been in that half hour, they still emerge, at the end of each episode, with renewed dignity and hope. When Ralph and Alice kiss and make up, as they inevitably do, we feel that all's right with the world. Like honeymooners everywhere, they—and we—are ready to start fresh and begin again.

No two people can live together, day in and day out, through stress and sickness and children and worries and family squabbles and every other human weakness and travail, and not expect to feel conflicted or estranged, used or alienated at one time or another. But the miracle of marriage, the miracle you have in each other, is that its strength is renewable. The two of you can always begin again. As long as you have the will, you can kiss and make up, forgive and forget, and keep on going, just like Ralph and Alice.

Each time a couple begins again, whether after an argument or after a crisis or just after a long week, their faith in each other is restored and their hope for the future is reaffirmed. They are a couple renewed with the spirit of honeymooners, the spirit that keeps them together and moves them from one landmark, one anniversary, one loving moment to the next.

৵৵৵ *DO YOU SEE YOURSELF HERE?* ৵৵৵

You may not see yourself here yet because you haven't been married that long, but we'll anticipate the questions so you can anticipate the delights you have ahead.

- Have you begun to notice how some longer-married couples relate to each other, how some seem more affectionate, more in love?
- Do you wonder if the two of you will be that way?
- Are you conscious of the signs and symbols of your love?
- Do you cultivate special moments and make them an occasion of celebration between you?
- Do you look forward to your anniversaries and try to make them extra special?
- Have you already thought about reaffirming your vows at some point in the future?
- Do you long for a second honeymoon (or maybe the first one you never took)?

The Look of Love

They have been married for over 50 years. She is a poet, who still writes and publishes, and he is a dentist, who still practices, although in a limited way. Every evening they can be seen taking their daily walk together, always hand in hand, swinging their arms, stopping to laugh, sometimes to hug. The way they talk, they way they move, the way they look at each other, it's obvious they're in love.

How is it that some couples exude such intimacy, such happiness? A gentle touch, a small caress, a knowing smile, these are the gestures of love. An unexpected gift, a small bouquet of flowers, an anniversary ring, these are the symbols. A special song, a secret code, a mealtime prayer of thanksgiving, these are the rituals. The gestures, symbols, and rituals of love, most so simple, but with effects so profound, because they remind us of why we married in the first place, and they reinforce those reasons along the way.

Every day, when the two of you choose to come home to each other, you are making a commitment to the marriage all over again. The homecoming, itself, is reason enough to rejoice; yet, how many couples don't even kiss when they're reunited after a long day? It doesn't mean, necessarily, that they've fallen out of love, but they are falling out of affection, and that's dangerous. That portends taking each other for granted.

As newlyweds, you're no doubt still conscious of the importance of small moments and sentimental gestures and try to make the most of them. Keep it up. The honeymoon is over when you start to forget; the marriage is over when you start not to care that you forgot.

Wedding Anniversaries

"We took a cruise for our honeymoon," says Iris. "We couldn't afford to do that again just a year later, so Josef booked us on a river cruise for dinner on our first anniversary. It was so romantic, and a real surprise, because he wouldn't tell me what we were doing, except to say that we were going to find the moonlight."

"Going to find the moonlight." What a perfect metaphor for the mood of anniversary celebrations. Whether it's your first, or your fifth, or your fifteenth, every anniversary is really special because it marks another year of love and commitment.

Here are some ideas for "finding the moonlight," even during the daytime, on your special date:

- Take the day off from work and do something really unusual, like going for a hot-air balloon ride, or renting a sailboat for a day. Whatever it is, it should be fun, romantic, and different.
- Call each other at work to say "I do" again at the exact time you exchanged vows. (Don't forget to allow for a different time zone if you were married in another location.)
- Write a poem, paint a picture, make your own greeting card. If you need a little help, go to a card shop that has computer assistance for making personalized cards.
- Make your anniversary gift instead of buying it. If you sew, or knit, or do woodwork, it should be easy, and you can make it out of one of the traditional materials for that year. (See next section under gifts.)
- Try to plan your yearly vacation over your anniversary date, if possible. That way, you'll always be somewhere new and exciting for your special day.
- Take pictures of yourselves each year so you can build a photographic history of your togetherness.
- Start saving a couple months in advance so you can really splurge for your anniversary: a limousine, dinner at an elegant restaurant, an evening at a supper club, orchestra seats at the theater or opera, maybe even an overnight stay at a five-star hotel. Indulge yourselves.
- Use an anniversary that falls on a weekend as an excuse for a getaway to the country or the seashore. Think of it as a mini-honeymoon.
- Do something crazy, like sending him a singing telegram or a balloon-o-gram at the office. By the way, you can send a man flowers, too.
- Display all the cards you get from friends and family, along with your wedding portrait or photo album, on your coffee table. The reminders will make your special day last a little longer.
- Agree to give each other one big gift for the home, then spend your anniversary shopping for it together.
- Decorate your dinner table in your wedding colors. If you celebrate at home, go through your wedding album over cocktails, and don't forget to have the top tier of your wedding cake for dessert, if it's your first anniversary. If it isn't, consider buying a mini-wedding-cake replica at the bakery, or make one and decorate it yourself.

- Make sure you toast each other and restate your commitment at whatever type of celebration you have. Besides the signs and the symbols, the words of love are important, too.

Anniversary Gift Giving

As mentioned under celebration suggestions, many couples reserve their anniversaries for giving each other gifts for the home, perhaps a stereo or a piece of furniture, something they both want and will enjoy. Sometimes, couples consider their anniversary celebration, the dinner out or the weekend getaway, as their gift to themselves, maybe presenting each other with only some small token or humorous remembrance as individual gifts. And then, of course, there are the biggies, the anniversaries that, for whatever reason, are so special as to warrant a serious piece of jewelry or a sensational second honeymoon.

A gift given with love and thoughtfulness is always wonderful, and yours to each other don't have to be large or lavish to be special. Creativity counts more than cost and, if you think about it for a while, you can no doubt come up with some original, memorable gift-giving ideas. You might even interpret the traditional, symbolic gifts (see list) in imaginative ways. For instance, for the first anniversary, paper could be anything from a box of stationery, to a newspaper subscription, to a trip to the Pacific Northwest to see a paper mill!

Relatives and friends, particularly close ones, will want to remember your anniversaries, too, and why shouldn't you let them share in your happiness? This is a good time to remind them of your bridal gift registry, especially if there are still items on that registry that you need to complete your home. Don't forget to write prompt thank-you notes for whatever gifts you receive.

There's a long-standing tradition for giving certain types of products as gifts for certain anniversaries, and that list follows. You'll often see a more contemporary version of this list in stores or other books, using plastic instead of paper, for example, or textiles instead of lace, presumably because some of the traditional items have become difficult, or expensive, to obtain. As always, you're

Traditional Anniversary Gifts

1. paper	9. pottery	25. silver
2. cotton	10. tin or aluminum	30. pearls
3. leather	11. steel	35. coral or jade
4. silk	12. linens (for tables, beds)	40. rubies
5. wood	13. lace	45. sapphires
6. iron	14. ivory	50. gold
7. wool	15. crystal	55. emeralds
8. bronze	20. china	60. diamonds

free to interpret tradition however you wish, even to create your own. The best gift is always the one that is most wanted and most appropriate for the person you have in mind.

Anniversary Parties

Some years you may want to celebrate quietly, privately and romantically, just the two of you. Other years, you may want to party. Then again, if you're lucky, you may even get to do both. That's what happened to one newlywed couple who celebrated their first anniversary at home, then flew across the country to visit his parents shortly thereafter, and were surprised with a big first-anniversary party there. "Really, it was more of a belated wedding reception, because most of Al's family and friends had not been able to attend our wedding," Lyssa explains. "But his parents called it an anniversary party, and it was great. Now we have twice as many memories of our first anniversary together."

There are all kinds of ways to celebrate, and all kinds of parties, too. Often, couples will simply have a few close friends or family members over to dinner. You might like to plan a casual buffet or barbecue, or even throw a big bash, and not tell anybody why. If you have friends with anniversaries around the same date as yours, you might decide it would be fun to celebrate together, either at home or with a night out on the town.

Except for landmark anniversaries or surprise parties, couples generally plan their celebrations themselves, so don't feel awkward about doing that. If you don't want gifts, then don't call your get-together an anniversary party, at least not until everyone has arrived.

Finally, if you're just looking for an excuse to have a party, especially a private party for just the two of you, don't overlook the other kinds of anniversaries you can celebrate. What about the anniversary of your first meeting, first date, first kiss, or even your first argument? Better yet, how about doing something special to celebrate the day you got engaged? Any excuse is a good one for establishing a history together.

Reaffirmation Ceremonies

A reaffirmation is a reenactment of your wedding vows. It is not another wedding and it does not involve any legalities, since you are already married, but it is a public recommitment to each other, whether that public is a large gathering, a religious congregation, or just a few close family and friends. You may choose to do this at any time for any reason, but usually couples wait for a "landmark" anniversary, fifth, tenth, or twenty-fifth, or have some special reason for choosing a particular year for the spiritual renewal reaffirmation brings.

The ritual of publicly renewing your marriage vows is more than just silly sentimentality, as increasing numbers of churches are recognizing with regular monthly anniversary services and group reaffirmations available to couples every year. As with the marriage ceremony itself, the ritual of reaffirmation repeats the words and reminds us of the promise we made to love and honor till death. There is something undeniably restorative for a couple in that act, especially when many years have passed or if the years have been particularly difficult.

With Style and Grace

Reaffirmation ceremonies can be as formal or as informal as you like, with or without a celebrant, religious or civil. Some couples do use the occasion to have the religious ceremony they didn't have the first time, and so renew their vows formally in a church or synagogue with friends and attendants present. Other couples might have the clergy or a civil officiant at home with a gathering of friends and renew their vows informally. Still others might write their recommitment pledges themselves, and exchange them casually among family and friends. Whatever the couple wants to do and is comfortable doing is entirely appropriate for them.

What you generally don't do is fully replicate the wedding, complete with matching bridesmaids, a wedding gown with a 50-foot train, and someone giving you away. (Entering with your husband is most appropriate.)

If your reaffirmation is to be a more formal affair held in a house of worship, then you and your husband will dress accordingly, even black tie if you prefer. You might choose to wear an off-white or pale pastel gown, with a corsage or carrying a single blossom instead of a bouquet. You may have honor attendants if you like (it's lovely if they can be the same people who attended you before), and don't forget to plan music and flowers to enhance the ceremony.

Talk to the clergy or officiant and see what he or she recommends. Even with a more formal ceremony, couples often personalize their vows. If your ceremony is less formal and/or being held at home, which seems somehow especially appropriate for a married couple, then you will have even more latitude in planning the kind of ceremony and reception you'd like to have. And if you have small children, don't forget to devise special roles for them in the festivities.

Yes, you read it correctly: it did say "ceremony" and "reception." Certainly, when you invite family and friends to share your renewal with you, you'll want to at least have champagne or another festive beverage and a "wedding cake" for the special event. You can also plan whatever other food and fare you think everyone would enjoy. If you have your reception at home, however, do get help for cooking and serving. After all, this is your celebration and you want to enjoy it!

Reaffirmation Invitations

Generally, a couple hosts their own reaffirmation ceremony and celebration, unless grown children are doing it for them. The choice of invitations should reflect the degree of formality of the affair and can range from the dignity of black ink engraved or thermographed on white stock to the informality of a phone call. Whatever suits your style best will be suitable to the occasion.

Wording for a very formal invitation reads very much like that for a wedding, except that the couple is hosting:

The honour of your presence (if religious)
or
The pleasure of your company (if not)
is requested at the reaffirmation
of the wedding vows of
Mr. and Mrs. John Smith
on Saturday, the nineteenth of July
nineteen hundred and ninety ___
at six o'clock
St. Leo Church
Roxbury Road
Reception immediately following
Candlelight Country Club
41 Club Road
R.S.V.P.   Black Tie

If the ceremony is informal, your invitation might read something like this:

John and Nancy Smith
cordially invite you to
the celebration of
the reaffirmation of their wedding vows
*on Saturday, July 19, 199_*
at 6 p.m.
at their home
124 Foxwood Road
Dinner following.
R.S.V.P.   No gifts please.

If the family or children of the couple are hosting the celebration, the invitation would read something like this:

The Smith family
request the pleasure of your company
at the reaffirmation of the wedding vows of
John and Nancy Smith
*on Saturday, July 19, 199_*
at 6 p.m.
at the Smith home
124 Foxwood Road.
Dinner following.
R.S.V.P.
Sally Smith Foster
000-000-0000

Ten Good Reasons
to Have a Reaffirmation Ceremony

1. Because your first wedding was a disaster.
2. Because your parents had the first one their way.
3. Because you couldn't afford the kind of wedding you wanted the first time.
4. Because your first wedding was too big, too formal, and no fun.
5. Because you had a civil ceremony, and now you want a religious one.
6. Because you've triumphed over a personal tragedy or trauma.
7. Because you want to doubly bless and celebrate another big event in your life: the birth of a baby, the christening of a new home, the launching of a new enterprise, etc.
8. Because your parents, siblings, or friends are also celebrating an important anniversary and want all of you to celebrate together.
9. Because there's some personal, sentimental reason for celebrating this anniversary in a special way.
10. Because you want to!

Note these differences between these invitations and wedding invitations: When you are hosting yourselves, it is perfectly appropriate to request "No gifts please." (You can also circulate the word that you would prefer gifts to charity if guests insist on giving.) If the invitation is formal, however, or if family is hosting for you, it is better not to stipulate no gifts, lest those guests who don't honor the request embarrass those who do.

Presumably, those you invite know you very well. So, when you are hosting, it is not necessary to give details of the addresses or a phone number for the response. When someone else is hosting, however, the response name and number needs to be stated.

The less formal the affair, the more license you can take with the wording and styling of the invitations. You may handwrite them, have blank cards calligraphied by machine, buy preprinted invitations and fill them in, or make them on a computer. If your affair is going to be fun and informal, you might even consider a "thematic" invitation reflecting your interests or professions, such as a notice of "renewal of the contract" for two married lawyers.

Savoring Second Honeymoons

"I honestly think our second honeymoon to the Caribbean [taken on the couple's fifth anniversary] was better than the first," says Marge of their trip to the Cayman Islands for scuba diving. "We looked forward to it for itself, not as an extension of the wedding, we were not tired and nervous, and we planned the trip together around an interest that's become a passion for us both. We're going to take another second honeymoon, as soon as we can afford it."

We've come full circle, back to where the discussion in this book began, only this time, when couples talk about their second honeymoons, their assessments are overwhelmingly positive. In fact, some couples like them so much they take them every year!

These days, second honeymoons are more common, and more frequent, because travel, even to exotic locations, has become more routine for most people than it used to be. Even so, the average couple probably can't afford an elaborate vacation each and every year, so they'll often save up for that special trip and then use it as a way to celebrate an anniversary or other life event. Any big trip that you designate as a second honeymoon, then, can be one.

But then there's the SECOND HONEYMOON, the ritualistic pilgrimage back to the same, original honeymoon destination, maybe even to the same identical hotel and the same identical suite. With luck, five, ten, fifteen, or twenty years later, you'll even find the same maitre d' or bartender in attendance, and he'll remember you as a young couple in love!

And that's how you'll remember yourselves as you begin to unwind and to feel transported back in time. Place can be powerfully sensual and evocative, especially when the associations with it are positive. The more you reenact the kinds of things you did together on your first honeymoon, the mountain hikes and midnight swims, the souvenir shopping and breakfast in bed, the more you'll rediscover who you are to each other.

These SECOND HONEYMOONS, intended to revive and recapture the romance of the original, deserve to be written in capital letters because they are special, indeed. And, in many ways, they are better than the first, because you are better, surer, more mature in your love. SECOND HONEYMOONS like these are usually reserved for the celebration of a landmark anniversary, often the tenth or twentieth, and they are made all the more delicious by the intervention of the years.

Ways to Save While You Savor

The one thing you're sure to notice as you return to your favorite destinations is the increased cost since your last visit—even if that visit was only a couple of years ago.

Ironically, for most popular resort areas, the cost of getting there has gone down, but the cost of staying there has risen. Try these strategies for helping your wallet match your memories.

- Ask about discounts. Often, you won't get them unless you do ask. Investigate "honeymoon packages" for second honeymooners, and tell them if you did, in fact, spend your honeymoon there. Some places, not many but some, will at least offer upgrades to returning guests.

- If your wedding was in peak season at your honeymoon location, consider taking your second honeymoon in the off season of the year. True, you won't be able to celebrate your actual anniversary at your destination, but you'll be able to afford to stay longer. Think about that.
- Use a travel agent, even if you know where you want to stay and exactly what you want to do. An agent is more knowledgeable about price breaks, discount fares, and the other ins and outs of package deals, so can usually get you the same accommodations you'd book yourself for less than it would cost you to do it.
- Don't relinquish your dream destination. In the interest of economy, look for ways to cut back without cutting out: a smaller room or one with a lesser view, a compact rental car, fewer tours or activities, less shopping, fewer elegant dinners, or a shorter stay.

What Other (Longer-Married) Couples Say . . .

You have much to look forward to, because the best is yet to come.

APPENDIX

As indicated in corresponding chapters, the following resources offer additional materials and information for interested readers.

Chapter 2: Establishing Your Couplehood

The Association for Couples in Marriage Enrichment (A.C.M.E.) is a non-profit, nonsectarian organization that promotes opportunities and resources that strengthen couple relationships and enhance personal growth, mutual fulfillment, and family wellness.

For a free catalogue of publications and more information about A.C.M.E. or A.C.M.E. events, write or call:

A.C.M.E.
Box 10596
Winston-Salem, NC 27108
(800) 634-8325

For a subscription to *Dovetail:* A Newsletter By and For Jewish–Christian Families, contact:

Dovetail Publishing
3014A Folsom Street
Boulder, CO 80304
(303) 444-8713
Joan C. Hawxhurst, Editor

The Intermarriage Handbook: A Guide for Jews and Christians, by Judy Petsonk and Jim Remsen (William Morrow/Quill Paperbacks, 1988), is a comprehensive guide for interfaith families.

"Only Love: A Guide to Happy Marriage" is a video for couples of all faiths. Created by Rev. Mark Connolly and narrated by Joe Garagiola, it is available for $39.95. Contact:

Rev. Mark Connolly
c/o Clemons Productions Inc.
Box 7466
Greenwich, CT 06830
(203) 869-9141

Chapter 4: Dealing with In-Laws

To learn more about an interfaith community, contact:

> Rabbi Charles Familant
> The Interfaith Community
> 332 O'Connor Street
> Menlo Park, CA 94025
> (415) 326-5330

For additional resources for interracial families, and a subscription to *New People,* a magazine for interracial couples ($15/year, $28/two years), contact:

> *New People*
> P.O. Box 47490
> Oak Park, MI 48237
> Yvette Walker Hollis, Editor

Chapter 5: Cultivating Intimacy

For a referral list of certified therapists in your area, contact:

> American Association of Sex Educators, Counselors,
> and Therapists (AASECT)
> 435 N. Michigan Avenue, Suite 1717
> Chicago, IL. 60611
> (312) 644-0828

The Better Sex Video Series written by Dr. Judy Seifer, is available for $29.95 plus postage and handling. Contact:

> The Townsend Institute
> Dept ZT12
> P.O. Box 8855
> Chapel Hill, NC 27515
> (800) 888-1900

For brochures and fact sheets on impotence, and for membership referral, contact:

> The Impotence Institute of America
> 2020 Pennsylvania Avenue N.W.
> Washington, D.C. 20006
> (800) 669-1603

Postponing Parenthood: The Effect of Age on Reproductive Potential, by Gale A. Sloan, R.N. (Plenum Press, 1993), $26.50. Can be ordered by calling:
(800) 221-9369

Chapter 6: Making a Home

Haven, a guide to planning a comfortable home, is offered by the Home Furnishings Council through member retailers. For the store nearest you offering free copies of *Haven,* call:

(800) 521-HOME, ext. 342

Quick Planner kits for Home, Kitchen, Bathroom, Office, and Interior Design are $15.95 each, plus $4 shipping and handling. To order, specify which kit and send a check or money order to:

H.M. Specialties
Dept HFQK 073
P.O. Box 1764
Sandusky, OH 44871-1764

For the Pier 1 store nearest you, or to be put on their mailing list, call:

(800) 447-4371

For a complete list of free or low-cost booklets on an incredibly broad range of topics researched by the U.S. Consumer Information Center, write to:

Consumer Information Catalog
Pueblo, CO 81009

Chapter 8: Managing Your Money: Short-Term Solutions

For brochures and information on handling credit, as well as the location of counseling offices in your area, contact:

Consumer Credit Counseling Service
8611 Second Avenue, Suite 100
Silver Springs, MD 20910
(800) 388-2227

For booklets on how to choose a financial planner, an interview sheet, a list of member financial planners in your area, and/or a copy of the "Financial Planning Consumer Bill of Rights: A Consumer Guide to Financial Independence," call:

International Association for Financial Planning
(800) 945-IAFP

For a referral list of three Certified Financial Planners in your area, call:

Institute of Certified Financial Planners
(800) 282-7526

Chapter 9: Building Financial Security: Long-Term Goals

For a home inventory guide, see your insurance agent or send a self-addressed, stamped business envelope to:

National Association of Professional Insurance Agents (PIA National)
400 N. Washington Street
Alexandria, VA 22314

Chapter 10: Understanding the Law

Terry J. Barnett. *Living Wills and More: Everything You Need To Ensure That All Your Medical Wishes Are Followed.* (John Wiley & Sons, 1992), $16.95. Contains model documents and instructions for every state.

For more information about agency adoptions, contact:

Child Welfare League of America
440 First Street N.W., Suite 310
Washington, D.C. 20001
(202) 638-2952

Also: National Committee for Adoption

1930 17th Street N.W.
Washington, D.C. 20009
(202) 328-1200

For emergency help in domestic abuse and referrals to shelters and safe houses in your area, call:

National Domestic Violence Hot Line
(800) 333-SAFE

For a list of publications on women's issues, including the comprehensive "State-by-State Guide to Women's Legal Rights" ($12.95 plus $2 postage), contact:

National Organization for Women
Legal Defense and Education Fund
99 Hudson Street
New York, NY 10013

The Public Education Division of the American Bar Association publishes many informative booklets available at low cost. Among them are:

"The American Lawyer: When and How to Use One"
(Publication #235-00021; $2.50 plus $2 postage and handling)

"Your Legal Guide to Marriage and Other Relationships"
(Publication #235-0005; $2.50 plus $2 postage and handling)

For these and/or a complete list of available publications, contact:

Order Fulfillment
American Bar Association
750 N. Lake Shore Drive
Chicago, IL 60611
(312) 988-5555

Chapter 11: Staying Healthy

The American Heart Association publishes numerous pamphlets on everything from restaurant dining to healthful recipes to exercise. For more information about their offerings, contact your local American Heart Association, listed in the white pages of the phone directory, or call:

(800) AHA-8721

For the list of brochures and information on various dental-care topics, contact:

The American Dental Association
211 E. Chicago Avenue
Chicago, IL 60611

For a free pamphlet, "Sunglasses Are More Than Shades," write:

American Optometric Association
243 N. Lindberg Blvd.
St. Louis, MO 63141

For a copy of a free brochure, "Choosing Your Physician: A Guide to Getting Quality Health Care," write:

The American Medical Association
515 N. State Street
Chicago, IL 60610

For more information about mental illness and free brochures on 18 different illnesses and disorders, write:

American Psychiatric Association
Division of Public Affairs
Department SHD
1400 K Street N.W.
Washington, D.C. 20005

REFERENCE NOTES

American Bar Association. *You and the Law.* Lincolnwood, Illinois: Publications International, Ltd., 1990.

Barnett, Terry J. *Living Wills and More.* New York: John Wiley & Sons, Inc., 1992.

Barringer, Felicity. "Census Bureau Places Population at 249.6 Million." *The New York Times,* 27 December 1990, B6.

Blair, Sampson Lee, and Michael P. Johnson. "Wives' Perceptions of the Fairness of the Division of Household Labor: The Intersection of Housework and Ideology." *Journal of Marriage and the Family,* 54, No. 3 (August 1992), 570–81.

Cahners Research. *Modern Bride's Consumer Council Survey: A Study of Newlywed Women.* New York: Cahners Publishing Company, July, 1993.

Cahners Research. *Modern Bride's Consumer Council: A Study of Engaged Women.* New York: Cahners Publishing Company, September, 1992.

Cahners Research. *Modern Bride's Consumer Council Survey: A Study of Newlywed Women.* New York: Cahners Publishing Company, March, 1992.

Chadwick, Bruce A., and Tim B. Heaton, eds. *Statistical Handbook on the American Family.* Phoenix: The Oryx Press, 1992.

Connidis, Ingrid Arnet. "Life Transitions and the Adult Sibling Tie: A Qualitative Study." *Journal of Marriage and the Family,* 54, No. 4 (November 1992), 972–82.

Crohan, Susan E., and Joseph Veroff. "Dimensions of Marital Well-being among White and Black Newlyweds." *Journal of Marriage and the Family,* 51, No. 2 (May 1989), 373–83.

Donovan, Patricia. *Testing Positive: Sexually Transmitted Disease and the Public Health Response.* New York: The Alan Guttmacher Institute, 1993.

Gibran, Kahil. *The Prophet.* New York: Alfred A. Knopf, 1966.

Greeley, Andrew. *Faithful Attraction: Discovering Intimacy, Love, and Fidelity in American Marriage.* New York: Tor Books, 1991.

Harlap, Susan, Kathryn Kost, and Jacqueline Darroch Forrest. *Preventing Pregnancy, Protecting Health: A New Look at Birth Control Choices in the United States.* New York: The Alan Guttmacher Institute, 1991.

Hochschild, Arlie, with Anne Machung. *The Second Shift: Working Parents and the Revolution at Home.* New York: Viking, 1989.

Klassen, Albert D., Colin J. Williams, and Eugene D. Levitt. *Sex and Morality in the U.S.: An Empirical Enquiry under the Auspices of The Kinsey Institute.* Middletown, Connecticut: Wesleyan University Press, 1989.

Kosmin, Barry, director. "The National Study of Religious Identification." City University of New York Graduate School, 1989–90.

Kurdek, Lawrence A. "Social Support and Psychological Distress in First-Married and Remarried Newlywed Husbands and Wives." *Journal of Marriage and the Family,* 51, No. 4 (November 1989), 1047–52.

Leder, Jane Mersky. "Adult Sibling Rivalry." *Psychology Today,* Jan./Feb. 1993, 56–60, 88–93.

McGoldrick, Monica, and Randy Gerson. *Genograms in Family Assessment.* New York: W.W. Norton & Company, 1985.

Money, John, M.D. *Love Maps: Clinical Concepts of Sexual/Erotic Health and Pathology, Paraphilia, and Gender Transposition in Childhood, Adolescence, and Maturity.* Buffalo, New York: Prometheus Books, 1988.

Pines, Ayala M., Ph.D. "Romantic Jealousy: The Shadow of Love." *Psychology Today,* Mar./Apr. 1992, 48–55.

Postman, Andrew. "What surprises men most about marriage." *Glamour,* May 1992, 214–17, 277.

Roberts, Thomas W. "Sexual Attraction and Romantic Love: Forgotten Variables in Marital Therapy." *Journal of Marital and Family Therapy,* 18, No. 4 (October 1992), 357–64.

Schoen, Robert. "First Unions and the Stability of First Marriages." *Journal of Marriage and the Family,* 54, No. 2 (May 1992), 281–84.

Simring, Sue Klavans, D.S.W., and Steven S. Simring, M.D., with William Proctor. "The Making of A Durable Marriage," *The Compatibility Quotient.* New York: Fawcett Columbine, 1990, 49–51.

Sloan, Gale A., R.N. *Postponing Parenthood: The Effect of Age on Reproductive Potential.* New York: Plenum Press, 1993.

Tenlin, Jon. "Why Women Are Mad as Hell." *Glamour,* March 1992, 206–9, 265–66.

Thomson, Elizabeth, and Ugo Colella. "Cohabitation and Marital Stability: Quality or Commitment?" *Journal of Marriage and the Family,* 54, No. 2 (May 1992), 259–67.

The Wall Street Journal. "People Patterns: Many Households Live Without Pocket Money," 6 August 1993, B1.

INDEX